HEALTH INEQUALITIES AND GLOBAL JUSTICE

HEALTH INEQUALITIES AND GLOBAL JUSTICE

Edited by Patti Tamara Lenard and
Christine Straehle

EDINBURGH
University Press

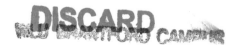

© editorial matter and organisation, Patti Tamara Lenard
and Christine Straehle, 2012
© the chapters their several authors, 2012

Edinburgh University Press Ltd
22 George Square, Edinburgh EH8 9LF
www.euppublishing.com

Typeset in 11/13 Palatino Light by
Servis Filmsetting Ltd, Stockport, Cheshire, and
printed and bound in the United States of America
by Edwards Brothers Malloy, Inc.

A CIP record for this book is available from the British Library

ISBN 978 0 7486 4692 0 (hardback)
ISBN 978 0 7486 4693 7 (webready PDF)
ISBN 978 0 7486 5652 3 (epub)
ISBN 978 0 7486 5651 6 (Amazon ebook)

The right of the contributors to be identified as authors of this work
has been asserted in accordance with the Copyright, Designs and
Patents Act 1988.

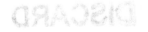

CONTENTS

ACKNOWLEDGEMENTS

We would like to thank the International Studies Association for its support in funding the workshop that gave rise to this volume. In particular, we would like to thank Marijke Breuning, who assisted us in the initial stages of the thematic planning, and Jeanne White, who shepherded us through the administrative side of organising such a workshop. Most importantly, we would like to thank Catherine Lu, who encouraged us to pursue this project, by applying to have it included in the ISA programme. We would also like to thank Jacob Levy for hosting the workshop at McGill University, and for providing us with logistical assistance in its preparation.

Special thanks are due to the editors at Edinburgh University Press, who have been tremendously supportive of this project from its inception. We'd like to thank Nicola Ramsey for her invaluable help in particular, in this regard. Thom Brooks, series editor for Global Justice Studies, has been enthusiastic about this project from the beginning, and has offered sage and calm advice as it has moved forward.

At the workshop itself, several friends and colleagues were gracious enough to offer comments on the papers delivered, and can take considerable credit for the high-quality chapters that appear in this volume: Anna Drake, Pierre-Yves Néron and Sarah Wiebe. We would also like to thank Cathy Nguyen and Katherine Wood for their excellent 'rapportage' of the day's events. We owe a special thanks to Katherine who, with good cheer, took responsibility for the tedious but critical job of formatting the manuscript for final submission.

Patti Tamara Lenard
Christine Straehle

NOTES ON THE CONTRIBUTORS

Yukiko Asada is Associate Professor in the Department of Community Health and Epidemiology at Dalhousie University. She is the author of *Health Inequality: Morality and Measurement* (2007). Her work investigates ethical assumptions underlying quantitative methods used in population health.

Gillian Brock is Associate Professor in the Philosophy Department at the University of Auckland. She has written extensively on issues of global justice. She is the author of *Global Justice: A Cosmopolitan Account* (2009) and editor or co-editor of *Current Debates in Global Justice* (2005), *The Political Philosophy of Cosmopolitanism* (2005), *Necessary Goods: Our Responsibilities to Meet Others' Needs* (1998) and *Global Health and Global Health Ethics* (2011).

Garrett Wallace Brown is Senior Lecturer in Political Theory and Global Ethics in the Department of Politics, University of Sheffield. His publications include work on cosmopolitanism, globalisation, global justice and global health governance. He has recently published *Grounding Cosmopolitanism* (Edinburgh University Press, 2009) and *The Cosmopolitanism Reader* (2010), and is currently publishing *Global Health Policy*.

Ryoa Chung is Associate Professor at the Department of Philosophy of the Université de Montréal. Her work published in English has appeared in *Critical Review of International Social and Political Philosophy*, *Public Health Ethics* and *Canadian Journal of Philosophy*. She is currently co-editing *Éthique des relations internationales* (forthcoming: 2013).

Phillip Cole has written on human rights and international migration, including the right to healthcare. His most recent work is *Debating the Ethics of Immigration: Is there a Right to Exclude?* (2011) with Christopher Heath Wellman. He is Visiting Professor in Applied Philosophy at Newport University, Wales.

Lisa Eckenwiler is Associate Professor of Philosophy in the Department of Philosophy at George Mason University. She also serves as Director of Health Ethics. Her current research focuses on ethical issues at the intersection of long-term care, health-worker migration and global health inequities. Her second book, *Long Term Care, Globalization, and Justice*, is forthcoming.

Nicole Hassoun is an Assistant Professor in Philosophy at Carnegie Mellon University. She is affiliated with Carnegie Mellon's Program on International Relations and the University of Pittsburgh's Center for Bioethics and Health Law. In 2009–10 she held a post-doctoral position at Stanford University and visited at the United Nations' World Institute for Development Economics Research. She has also been a visiting scholar at the Center for Poverty Research in Austria and the Center for Advanced Studies in Frankfurt. Her book, *Globalization and Global Justice: Shrinking Distance, Expanding Obligations*, is forthcoming.

Daniel M. Hausman is the Herbert A. Simon and Hilldale Professor of Philosophy at the University of Wisconsin-Madison. His research has centred on epistemological, metaphysical and ethical issues lying at the boundaries between economics and philosophy. His most recent book, just published, is *Preference, Value, Choice and Welfare*.

Matthew R. Hunt is an Assistant Professor in the School of Physical and Occupational Therapy and Affiliate Member of the Biomedical Ethics Unit at McGill University, Montreal. His research focuses on ethical issues related to two domains: global health engagement, and rehabilitation care and professions.

Angela Kaida is a global health epidemiologist interested in the linkages between HIV and reproductive health. She is a Canada Research Chair (Tier 2) in Global Perspectives in HIV and Sexual and Reproductive Health and an Assistant Professor in the Faculty of Health Sciences at Simon Fraser University.

Eszter Kollar is Adjunct Assistant Professor, International Affairs, John Cabot University, as well as a Research Fellow at the Center for Ethics and Global Politics/Faculty of Political Science, LUISS University, Rome. Before that, she held a post-doctoral fellowship at the Hoover Chair, Catholic University of Louvain. She is co-editor, with Miriam Ronzoni, of a symposium on Gillian Brock's *Global Justice: A Cosmopolitan Account – Global Justice: Theory Practice Rhetoric* (2010).

Patti Tamara Lenard is Assistant Professor of Applied Ethics at the Graduate School of Public and International Affairs, University of Ottawa. Her first book is *Trust, Democracy and Multicultural Challenges*.

Adina Preda is a research fellow in the Centre for Research in Ethics at the University of Montreal (CRÉUM), currently working on a collaborative project on health equity (M-HERC). Prior to this, she was a Hoover fellow at the Hoover Chair, Catholic University of Louvain and a lecturer in political theory at University College Dublin.

Christine Straehle is Assistant Professor of Applied Ethics at the Graduate School of Public and International Affairs, University of Ottawa.

Sridhar Venkatapuram is a Wellcome Trust Research Fellow in Ethics at the London School of Hygiene and Tropical Medicine, and an Affiliated Lecturer at Cambridge University. His current research is at the intersection of health sciences and social justice philosophy. His first monograph, *Health Justice: An Argument from the Capabilities Approach*, was published in 2011.

Kristin Voigt is a post-doctoral fellow at McGill University, jointly in the Department of Epidemiology, Biostatics and Occupational Health and the Biomedical Ethics Unit. Her research focuses on egalitarian theories of social justice and egalitarian concerns around health policy.

INTRODUCTION: HEALTH INEQUALITY AND GLOBAL REDISTRIBUTIVE JUSTICE

Patti Lenard and Christine Straehle

It is now frequently observed that millions around the world die from preventable diseases, and that millions more suffer from poor health as a result of extreme poverty. However 'health' is defined and however it is measured – and there is considerable controversy about both defining and measuring health – the citizens of developing countries fare significantly worse than citizens of developed countries: life expectancy ranges from 40 (in some sub-Saharan African countries) to over 80 (in many western, developed nations); the number of doctors ranges from fewer than 5 per 100,000 people to nearly 600 per 100,000 (in many sub-Saharan African countries, and in Cuba, respectively); health expenditure ranges from less than US$3 per person per year to over US$5,000 per year (in many sub-Saharan African countries, and in the USA, respectively); and the infant mortality rate ranges from 3/1,000 in Iceland to nearly 200/1,000 in Angola (World Health Organization 2007). These statistics, even if well-known, are startling, and reveal the depth of the differences in health outcomes for citizens around the world.

The causes of the appallingly poor health outcomes in developing nations are complex, to say the least, as are the difficulties we face in identifying who, if anybody, is responsible for them and who should take on the responsibility to remedy then. For many, among them several contributors to this volume, it is increasingly clear that poor health in the developing world is not only a local problem, but also a consequence of multiple global decisions, for example, to permit global patents on life-saving drugs and to permit morally egregious health-care-worker recruiting policies in the developing world. Fortunately, for those who live in developing nations, concerns about global health inequalities are increasingly a matter of political attention. For example,

1

Canada recently announced its intention to focus on maternal health in the developing world during its G8 presidency, the United Nations Millennium Development Goals (MDG) focus on improving health outcomes, and much political and public attention is being paid to the Bill and Melinda Gates Foundation's, and Warren Buffet's, efforts to improve the quality of health in the developing world. But despite such increased attention, the prospects for health in developing nations are grim: the 2015 MDG goals are unlikely to be met; the G8 emphasis on maternal mortality is fraught with ideological conflict in developed nations; and the contributions that are being made by health research foundations are significant, but not adequate to turn the tide of poor health outcomes in developing nations.

This volume focuses on the moral dilemmas posed by these evident health inequalities, and examines to what extent inequalities in health pose problems for those concerned with justice in general, and global justice in particular. The demands of global justice have been debated for some time now, and many have argued that any plausible account of global *in*justice takes its starting point from accounts of wealth inequalities and an analysis of why such inequalities are unjust. This volume's authors examine the extent to which global inequalities in health can be addressed as the product of global wealth inequalities more generally, or whether inequalities in health pose specific and distinct problems to moral and political philosophy, in particular at the global level.

Historically, political and moral philosophers have had little to say on the topic of health as a component of distributive justice (there are exceptions, of course, including Daniels 1981; Daniels 2008; Segall 2009; Venkatapuram 2011). When health has been addressed thus far, it has largely been so only in the context of rights. Scholars of human rights have sought to define the rights to which we are entitled by virtue of our humanity, and we have seen ongoing debate concerning whether the 'right to health', or the 'right to healthcare', should be considered a basic right (Mann 1996; Pogge 2005c; Nickels 2007). And while the United Nations Declaration on Human Rights includes the right to health on its list of basic human rights, it is more typically the case that the right to health is included in the category of 'social' rights, and social rights in general have not received the same attention in human rights debates as have political and civic rights (Shue 1996).

This 'rights' focus is an extraordinarily important one, as many of our authors suggest; but it falls short of addressing the fundamental inequalities in health, since a focus on rights as they have been framed so far suggests that our obligation is simply to refrain from violating them (Pogge 2002). In the view of many of the contributors here, however, the obligation of non-harm is inadequate, since it neglects the global economic institutions that affect health outcomes in many developing nations. These need to be analysed from a perspective that is more encompassing than 'rights', if our goal is to ensure justice in health (Gostin 2007). Thus, the contributions to our volume move beyond the rights debate, at least in its limited 'non-harm' form, to examine health inequalities in the context of global distributive inequalities, with the objective of pursuing global redistributive justice. In particular, four distinct conceptual questions, and one key empirical question, frame the contributions to this book:

1. What does a right to health entail?
2. How does this right connect to discussions of distributive justice?
3. Who bears responsibility for protecting the right to health?
4. Whose obligation is it to remedy health inequalities, in particular those that are the product of unjust wealth distribution across borders?
5. Once we have determined the content of the right to health, or of health equality, and the concomitant responsibilities, how can we measure whether a nation scores well or poorly in achieving these objectives?

These latter measurement questions are essential to determining where we need to focus our policies if our goal is to pursue 'health equality': is it in the domain of recruitment, or training of health professionals, for example, or simply in providing access to basic medical services, or elsewhere? These latter questions are tackled by the chapters featured in the final section of this volume.

PART 1: A RIGHT TO *EQUAL* HEALTH?

The first chapters of this book consider the notion of a right to health, in particular whether there is such a right, and if there is such a right, what it might entail, and once its content is defined, whether this right can be equalised in any meaningful way. These are enormously difficult questions.

One difficulty stems from the connections between good health and socio-economic indicators of wealth. Wealthy people are healthier; more educated people are healthier; individuals who live in physically secure environments are healthier. These correlations indicate, for some, that health outcomes are merely dependent on levels of wealth and education more generally. On this view, any standard attempt to 'equalise' wealth will thus 'equalise' health outcomes. If we educate people, if we provide them with sufficient income, and provide for social stability, health will improve without our focusing on it directly. According to this argument, health is a function of socio-economic redistribution; there is therefore no need for independent theorising on the content of the right to health and the duties we acquire in light of acknowledging it.

The fact that health correlates so well with indicators of socio-economic wealth suggests to some that 'health' is not a distinct category of well-being with which we should be independently concerned.[1] But this is a mistake. For one thing, health (merely) correlates with other indicators of wealth; yet, many wealthy people are not healthy (indeed, one of the negative effects of development is the spread of dangerous, *non-communicable*, diseases that correlate with increasing levels of wealth) and many poor people are healthy. It would also be a mistake to equate wealth with improved access to healthcare since evidence taken from around the world shows that citizens of some countries have better access to quality in healthcare than others (at comparable levels of wealth). Second, the conditions under which healthcare can be made accessible are not entirely dependent on (considerable) resources. The infrastructure on which healthcare delivery depends can be constructed and maintained even in relatively less affluent areas, so long as it is prioritised to some degree. It is then not enough simply to redistribute wealth across societies and assume that health inequalities will be therefore addressed. Instead it is important to think about an independent right to health and define the content such a right would have.

This definitional challenge, however, is accompanied by other challenges. For one, health is not something that we can guarantee, even if we try very hard and even if we can agree on a definition of what provisions health requires. Whether an individual is healthy is to a considerable degree a matter of luck, and there will be individuals for whom an infinite amount of healthcare will nevertheless fail to produce good health. We wouldn't like to say that a person for whom this kind of effort is expended, to no avail, is denied a reasonably defined right to health. There is, ultimately, an imperfect relationship between the right to health (when it is respected) and health outcomes: positive or negative health outcomes are not sufficient to indicate whether the right to health is being respected. This is an observation that Adina Preda makes in the opening chapter. It may make more sense, she suggests, to define the right to health in terms of *healthcare*. We should identify an appropriate standard of healthcare, where when met, we can conclude that the right to health is respected. Exceptions to whatever rule we determine will undoubtedly exist as well; just as the right of all citizens to access a publicly provided library can require that additional efforts are made to ensure that individuals with limited mobility can enter libraries, the right to a standard of healthcare may demand that additional efforts be made with respect to specific individuals.

Preda's chapter invites readers to consider, additionally, the connection between egalitarian political theory – much of which is concerned with the equal distribution of material resources – and the protection of a supposed right to equal health. Since, as we indicated above, we can never guarantee that a specific distribution of resources will produce equality in health outcomes, the precise application of egalitarian distributive theories of justice to questions of health – and in particular in protecting a supposed right to health – proves challenging, for reasons Preda explores.

In light of these challenges, Daniel M. Hausman rejects a strictly luck egalitarian approach to understanding the possible demands of a right to health. Luck egalitarianism tells us that our primary concern should be with neutralising the effects of bad luck – to the extent that our health status is a matter of luck, therefore, luck egalitarianism tells us that we should find ways to redistribute resources (in this case, access to healthcare) to those who are less healthy through no fault of their own. But, says Hausman, the luck egalitarian lens is too narrow: for example, it will tell us that we should be concerned to redistribute resources from Paraguay to Russia, since although Paraguay is considerably less wealthy than Russia, its health outcomes are considerably better. Instead, Hausman argues, we ought to take a 'relational' approach to understanding health inequalities: at the domestic level, a relational approach tells us that our central concern should be with whether individuals can interact with each other under conditions of equal respect; and at the global level, it tells us that to the extent that poor health impairs the capacity of a nation to interact with others on an equal basis, we should be concerned with redistributing resources to ensure equal access to healthcare across nations.

Taking a broadly relational approach focuses our attention on how others are doing, and how our ability to interact as equals depends on at least a minimal standard of health (among other things, evidently). Although framed differently, Lisa Eckenwiler's chapter also asks readers to take a relational view seriously; she terms her approach ecological, by which she means that we should understand ourselves and others as necessarily situated in specific places that determine the nature of our relationships. An ecological approach can draw our attention to how our identities are both 'intersubjectively constructed' and 'mutually constitutive'. The consequence of this emphasis will increase our understanding of our responsibility for others in general, and for their health outcomes in particular.

Whereas Hausman and Eckenwiler emphasise the ways in which we can best approach remedying health inequalities by focusing on the ways in which health outcomes are determined by human relations, Sridhar Venkatapuram and Phillip Cole both take a 'capabilities' approach to evaluating the dilemmas posed by health inequalities across borders. The capabilities approach in political theory self-consciously emphasises 'what people are actually able to do and be' and thus underlines 'health' as one among the capabilities that must be protected in order to secure human flourishing (Nussbaum 2000: 5; Nussbaum 2005). Furthermore, it emphasises the importance of protecting and promoting individuals' abilities to make decisions about their own lives and to pursue valuable objectives over the course of them. The capabilities approach thus differs from a traditional rights approach by analysing not only the rights to which individuals must have access, but also the use that individuals can actually make of their rights in their specific social contexts, as Ventakapuram explains. Applying the capabilities approach at the global level helps to shed light on the challenges posed by health inequalities within and across societies.

PART 2: WHO IS RESPONSIBLE FOR REMEDYING GLOBAL HEALTH INEQUALITY?

Although the authors who contribute to the 'rights' debate do not agree on the *justification* for defining and protecting a right to health in Part 1, none denies the moral dilemmas posed by the depth of inequalities in health across the world. And even though wealth is not the only determinant of health, strong inequalities in health divide citizens of the wealthiest nations from those in the poorest nations. Yet, locating the agents who are a) responsible for these inequalities and, more importantly perhaps, b) responsible to remedy these inequalities is by no means straightforward, as several of our authors indicate.

In the opening chapter to Part 2, Garrett Wallace Brown outlines three different ways in which we might respond to health inequalities. A 'lifeboat ethics' approach takes its central insight from Thomas Malthus' theories of population growth and argues that population growth would stall when resources became inadequate to support additional lives. This approach suggests that we ought to avoid extending aid to those who are suffering, on the idea that something like 'natural selection' is operating to sustain a manageable population. Aside from the cruelty associated with ignoring those in desperate need, this approach should be rejected for ignoring the extent to which our lives are influenced by the actions of those around us; Brown's critique thus echoes some of Eckenwiler and Hausman's concerns. Often, our health outcomes will be the result of actions taken by others, that we cannot control, rather than by 'nature' operating to protect the strongest among us. A second approach, the 'proximity approach', tells us that health inequality is problematic when it affects those nearest to us, that is, those who live within our national boundaries. On this view, although we should object to health inequalities within national boundaries, the health inequalities that divide health-rich from health-poor nations, though appalling, are not the responsibility of the wealthy. This view, says Brown, should equally be rejected, for violating a central intuition of much egalitarian political theory: that we should be held responsible only for what we can reasonably control. Those who are victims of poor health in developing nations find themselves in conditions they did not choose, and therefore they should not be held responsible for their health status. Instead, says Brown, and this is a view echoed in later chapters, we should adopt a cosmopolitan approach to health inequalities: on this view, our main concern should be with instantiating a commitment to the equal moral worth of all individuals. As applied to the domain of health, this requires intervening in developing nations in which the health conditions are poor, with the purpose of offering aid.

Gillian Brock expands on one dimension of a cosmopolitan approach to health inequalities. In her view, we have remedial responsibilities to come to the aid of those in need; remedial duties are those that we have simply in virtue of our capacity to carry them out. Wealthy nations have the capacity to come to the aid of those who are health-deprived, which for Brock demands a more expansive focus than on health specifically, and includes additionally a focus on the ways in which the global economic system operates to sustain the poverty and poor health outcomes of those in developing nations. Some thinkers aim to allocate responsibility for health inequalities by pointing to those who are responsible for causing poor health in others; although Brock does not dismiss this strategy, her goal is to identify the role that wealthy nations can play in effecting what she terms 'transitional justice', that is, a transition from what we have now, a world plagued by health inequalities, to something that is closer to an ideal, a world in which health inequalities are not so vast. Wealthy nations, she argues, ought to show moral leadership in the domain of health. Brock's chapter thus sets up the argument made by Angela Kaida and Patti Tamara Lenard. Kaida and Lenard's chapter articulates how cosmopolitan political principles point towards the conclusion that wealthy nations – because they have adequate resources, because they have demonstrated the capacity to do so in the past, and because they have made promises to do so – are obligated to continue to fight the HIV/AIDS epidemic in sub-Saharan Africa, in particular as this epidemic continues disproportionately to affect the lives of women and children. Such obligations can be assigned even in the absence of a clear definition of the right to health: even if we can't agree on the content of the right to health, we can certainly hold that it is violated if people die prematurely due to preventable, or treatable, diseases.

PART 3: MEASURING HEALTH OR HEALTH OUTCOMES

An analysis of the HIV/AIDS epidemic points to a related problem. If we take Kaida and Lenard's chapter to indicate that there is an obligation to provide healthcare to those affected by the disease, we will still need to define the measures of that care: we can measure, as evidence (or not) that the right is being respected, the number of doctors per capita; infant mortality; incidences of river blindness; life expectancy; and so on.

Kristin Voigt tackles the challenges of generating appropriate mechanisms by which to measure global health, in particular with a goal of articulating the imperative of designing health measures in ways that are normatively unproblematic. Health measures can, if designed poorly, lead to injustices in the ways in which resources are allocated, for example. In her chapter, Voigt evaluates the way in which this concern – about unjust resource allocation – has influenced researchers associated with the Global Burden of Disease study, who have relied on disability-adjusted life-years (DALYs) to quantify the disease burden around the world. The DALY measurement considers the number of life-years lost as a result of premature mortality, the number of years individuals live with a particular health condition, and the severity of this condition. Voigt aims in her chapter to assess the challenges faced by researchers concerned to develop a morally neutral measure of global health – a measure, that is, that respects the moral equality of all human beings described by Brown in their specific social contexts. The DALY measurement, if implemented well, can give us a genuine understanding of where health conditions are poor and are in need of remedy as a condition of achieving global justice in health.

Yukiko Asada takes her lead from the capabilities approach described above, and suggests we move towards a 'sufficiency' view – since health is a capability, we can interpret having adequate 'health capability' as having attained health sufficiency, an attainment which, if met globally, would satisfy our moral requirements with respect to remedying health inequalities. Says Asada, we can then measure whether sufficiency has been attained with respect to health via a 'health utilities index' (HUI), which measures an individual's functionality along eight dimensions (vision, hearing, speech, mobility, dexterity, emotion, cognition, pain) and converts these levels into a score based on social preferences of particular health states. Asada presents an example: 'The HUI score for a near-sighted but otherwise fully functional individual is 0.973, and this score reflects the average societal preference, rather than the respondent's assessment, of how good this particular health state is compared to full health' (pp. 164–5). We ought therefore to take the average HUI within a specific society as the measure of 'sufficiency', and aim to achieve that level of health within a society more generally.

This may help us unpack the question of responsibility for providing access to health, as framed by Nicole Hassoun. Hassoun's central concern is to find a way to motivate pharmaceutical companies to contribute their research expertise to remedying global diseases. Modelled on the fair trade movement more generally, she proposes developing a rating system which she terms the 'global health impact rating', where the drugs produced by pharmaceutical companies that have contributed to remedying global disease will be labelled as such. Consumers in western healthcare-rich nations (in particular) will therefore be able to make choices among companies according to their contribution to health equality around the world. In order to develop this rating system, of course, we require a robust mechanism by which to measure whether a given drug has served to save or extend lives. This measurement mechanism, says Hassoun, must consider three issues: how we identify what counts as a health need; how we measure drug effectiveness; and how we measure drug access. Hassoun's chapter makes positive proposals along each of these dimensions.

PART 4: BORDERS AND HEALTH

Of course we need not look across borders to witness health inequalities. Domestic political communities are often characterised by health inequalities, often pernicious ones. This observation frames Matthew R. Hunt and Ryoa Chung's chapter, which considers the intersection of existing health inequalities and humanitarian disasters. In cases of pre-existing health inequalities in a given community, the onset of a humanitarian disaster serves only to exacerbate these inequalities. Chung and Hunt propose we take what they term a 'structured vulnerabilities approach', according to which post-disaster aid workers must be attentive to the fact that some populations – those that are already disadvantaged prior to the disaster – are even more vulnerable following the disaster. Aid workers should focus not simply on providing aid to those who are most vulnerable; they should also focus on dismantling the social structures that restrict some populations to conditions of persistent vulnerability.

Phillip Cole also worries about health inequalities *within* borders. Cole considers whether there is any justification *within* a territory to distinguish among residents with respect to healthcare access. In Canada and the United States, for example, non-permanent residents are not permitted access to public healthcare beyond emergency services; in these countries, the different access is justified at least in part in terms of 'protecting' resources, by barring non-permanent residents from participation in a whole host of social services. For many, however, this distinction is unjust; all those who contribute meaningfully to the economy, whether permanent residents or not, should have access to the full range of social services. Cole considers an even more controversial question, whether *illegal* migrants should have access to health services in the country in which they reside. Cole argues that since healthcare is a right, and since it is a right that can be justified for its contribution to human flourishing and in its status as a basic capability, attempts to deny irregular migrants access to healthcare amount to a fundamental injustice. Just as, in Cole's view, there is no basis for distinguishing between insiders and outsiders, that is, people who live on different sides of borders, there is equally no moral basis for distinguishing between insiders and supposed outsiders who reside within shared, territorially delimited, boundaries.

If, as Cole and many other contributors to this volume suggest, borders should have no influence on any individual's right to healthcare, we may have good reason to worry about the migration of medical professionals from developing nations to developed nations. One common explanation given for poor health outcomes in developing nations is the inadequate access these citizens have to healthcare. Citizens across developing nations often do not have access to doctors and nurses, and these medical professionals are themselves often hampered by inadequate access to the resources they need to treat the ill. Medical professionals are additionally asked to labour in poor conditions and often, in particular, for little remuneration. In light of this and the challenges that developed nations are having in providing the standard of healthcare to which their own citizens have become accustomed, we see considerable movement of healthcare professionals from poor nations to wealthy nations. The result is a de facto subsidy of rich nations by poor nations: poor nations educate health professionals, who then migrate to put their education to use in wealthy nations, for considerably higher incomes. This is particularly problematic when such migration is prompted by aggressive recruitment by wealthy nations in poor nations.

We can evaluate this situation from the perspective of the health worker who chooses to migrate as well as from those left behind in developing nations. Together, Eszter Kollar's chapter and Christine Straehle's chapter consider the difficult normative issues that should inform responses to this form of migration. On the one hand, individuals – including those with valuable skills – should be permitted to exercise their right to migrate; Straehle emphasises the ways in which attempts to prevent the migration of health workers can, in most of their incarnations, violate their autonomy. On the other, says Kollar, the effect of the migration of health professionals renders the realisation of the human right to health impossible in developing nations. Kollar considers whether international law, which constrains movement in certain circumstances, some of which involve health (for example, migration is constrained when we are concerned with the spread of disease across borders), can serve to underpin restrictions on the movement of health professionals to prevent this human right violation; her analysis is inconclusive, however.

CONCLUSION

It is clear that there are profound inequalities that divide the healthiest from the least healthy members of our global community; and that these inequalities should give us moral pause. What is less clear is *what* the injustice is that is being perpetrated, who (if anyone) is perpetrating this injustice, and who is responsible for remedying this injustice. The chapters in this book tackle these difficult questions. Together, the authors attempt to identify a) the content of a positive right to health or to healthcare, b) the grounds on which the responsibility to protect this right can be attributed to specific actors, and c) the responsibilities these actors have for generating the best mechanisms by which this right can be protected. The challenges in tackling these tasks are exacerbated, as the contributors note, by the difficulties associated with *measuring* health inequalities: the measurement strategy we choose correlates heavily with the responsibilities that we assign and acknowledge.

Ultimately, the authors in this collection do not provide a unified answer to the difficult questions that motivated the collection initially.

They do, however, serve to highlight both the questions that must be asked and the range of factors that we ought to consider when answering them.

Note

1. For some discussion, see Hessler 2008: 31–43.

Part 1

A Right to *Equal* Health?

Chapter 1

IS THERE A HUMAN RIGHT TO HEALTH?[1]

Adina Preda

The International Covenant on Economic, Social and Cultural Rights (ICESCR) proclaims a universal human right to health, in Article 12, which reads:

> The States Parties to the present Covenant recognize the right of everyone to the enjoyment of the highest attainable standard of physical and mental health.

Let us briefly note some features of this right. First, this is a positive right that requires positive action on the part of corresponding duty bearers; the legal duties to fulfil this right fall primarily on one's state. Second, this is a right to the *enjoyment* of health, rather than a right to goods or services (such as healthcare) that would enable one to have a healthy life. In other words, it is a right to a certain *outcome* in terms of health and not merely to the opportunity for health. Third, it is a right to *the highest attainable standard* rather than an adequate or sufficient level of health. However, the highest attainable standard is normally interpreted in a rather conservative fashion, in the sense that it refers to the highest standard achievable in a specific country, given its resource limitations. This means that not all right-holders everywhere are entitled to the same level of health.

The question I want to address in this paper is whether this *legal* right is justified; in other words, whether there is a *moral* human right to health. I will proceed by asking two separate questions: first, whether an equal moral right to health, rather than healthcare or the provision of other goods, can be argued for, and second, whether this can be a universal human right. The chapter is structured as follows: in the first section, I clarify the notion of human rights and the way in which a right to a specific good can be justified. In the second and third sections, I examine a luck egalitarian and a Rawlsian account of justice in health respectively, and in the last section, I consider some specific challenges faced by positive rights, more specifically the idea that they cannot be general rights.

THE CONCEPT AND JUSTIFICATION OF HUMAN RIGHTS

According to the most common but still pertinent definition, human rights are the rights that all human beings possess simply in virtue of their humanity. In spite of its simplicity, this definition can point to some relevant features of human rights, of which I want to highlight two. First, a human right must be a *general* rather than a *special* right, if it is to be possessed by all human beings *simply in virtue of their humanity*. Having a general right does not depend on being a member of any particular society, contract or any other special relationship.[2] General rights are thus *pre-institutional* rights. Special rights, by contrast, are those that only a sub-set of humans possess in virtue of being part of a specific arrangement, contract or agreement, which broadly includes being part of a specific society or co-operative scheme. This further implies that, if no special institutional or societal arrangements need be in place in order for human rights to exist, they must be held against everyone else, rather than only people who are part of a particular institutional arrangement or scheme of co-operation. Human rights are thus rights held not only by all human beings but also *against all* other human beings.

This first condition implies that rights held against one's government or society are *citizens'* rather than human rights (Jones 1994: 86–90). So most positive human rights as currently interpreted by legal standards are not genuine human rights since they are rights against one's government. Thus, if the legal right to health is to have a moral counterpart, it must be possible to ascribe the first-order duties correlative to it to all other human beings. This is not to say that governments may not have *second-order* duties to enforce, protect and promote this right.

The second condition that a right must fulfil in order to count as a human right is that it must be an *equal* right. Since there are no qualifying conditions for holding human rights except being human, all human beings must have a right with the same content. This is not to say that these rights cannot be modified, or indeed enhanced as it were, in virtue of being part of a special relationship, but for a *human* right to exist it must be the same for everyone. Since it must be an equal right of all against all, the human right to health cannot be a right to a health status that differs from country to country, if it is to be a genuine human right. A genuine human right to health, if any, will give human beings everywhere a claim to the same level of health and everyone will also have a corresponding duty –at least in the first instance – to ensure that this level is achieved for everyone. If this is the case, the highest attainable level might be interpreted as the highest level currently attainable given the state of technology and global resources; but it is probably not feasible to aim for this level of health *for everyone*. So in what follows I will assume instead that the human right to health should be interpreted simply as a right to a *specified* but equal level of health and I will ask whether such a right can be justified.

There are generally two ways in which a right to a specific good can be justified: we can adopt a rights-based or a justice-based perspective. In other words, we can either start by trying to justify a particular right (generally on the basis of human needs, interests or agency) or we can start by arguing for principles of distributive justice, which may in turn generate certain rights. The former has been, perhaps naturally, more popular in the field of human rights, while the latter has not in fact paid special attention to rights. One of the aims of my paper is to argue that we should adopt the latter perspective while paying more attention to the way in which it can yield particular rights.

The literature on human rights is rife with arguments that purport to ground various moral rights. Although the rights perspective might be a natural candidate for a justification of a particular right, it suffers from incompleteness, particularly when it comes to positive rights. This is because genuine rights entail *correlative* duties; some duties are negative, that is, duties to refrain from interference with the object of the right. Other rights, like the right to health, correlate with positive duties, that is, duties to provide the right-holder with a good or service. In order to justify a positive right to X, it is not sufficient to show that human beings have an interest in X or that X is an important value; a suitable justification of a positive right must show that such duties can be legitimately imposed on others and that it is a duty that correlates to a right. Assuming that all (and only) duties of justice are correlative to rights, a suitable justification must show that justice requires the provision of such goods and services. Surprisingly, this is a requirement that is often neglected by theorists who adopt a perspective that focuses on rights.

It seems to me that, in order to justify a right, one should go beyond the framework of rights in the direction of a theory of distributive justice. For this reason, I will focus on how theories of distributive justice *can* ground a right to a specific good, in this case health. However, theories of justice, by contrast, have – again, perhaps surprisingly – not paid sufficient attention to rights. They tend to outline principles of justice which can yield certain requirements and perhaps policy prescriptions but they are often silent on the kinds of right that can be generated based on these. Yet it seems to me that this is a necessary step; if the purpose of a theory of justice is to construct principles that could be translated into law and since the law is a system of rules that confer rights, the purpose of a theory of justice should be able to generate a set of just rights.[3] Thus, in what follows, I attempt to fill this gap and see how some existing theories of justice in health could yield specific rights and in particular whether they can justify a right to health.

But let me first clarify what it takes for a theory of justice to generate a right to health. We established that a human right to health, if any, would be an equal right of all against all. Thus I take it that a theory of justice can justify a right to health just in case it can argue for equality in health *per se*, that is, equality in health outcomes. This is what I will refer to as a right to health *per se*, which may require the provision of unequal amounts of good or resources to individuals depending on their health needs. By contrast, I will use a right to health *care* to refer to a right to certain goods and services, which should in principle be provided equally to everyone. A separate question is whether such a right is a universal human right. In order to yield such a right, a theory of justice should argue for equality in health on a global level; in other words, it must be a cosmopolitan theory. But I will not examine this issue since a theory of justice might be cosmopolitan and yet institutional, so the rights it will generate will not be general, pre-institutional rights. I will instead examine at the end some preliminary, conceptual difficulties that positive rights might face.

So in order to find a justification for a right to health we need to look at egalitarian theories of justice in health. So far only two kinds of egalitarian theory of justice in health have been put forward: a luck egalitarian theory and a Rawlsian-inspired theory; so I will focus on the accounts provided by Shlomi Segall and Norman Daniels. I will show that neither of them can generate a right to equal outcomes in health, which is unsurprising given that this is not even their intention. Segall aims to argue for universal healthcare – hence a right to healthcare – but I will argue that he does not succeed, at least not within the confines of luck egalitarianism. The arguments he appeals to are independent of, and possibly inconsistent with, his luck egalitarian commitments. By contrast, Daniels' argument might support a right to an equal, albeit minimum, level of health in spite of the fact that he explicitly claims his account generates a right to both health and healthcare.

Luck Egalitarianism

The central thought of a luck egalitarian theory is that 'it is unfair for one person to be worse-off than another due to reasons beyond her control' (Segall 2010: 10). Now there may be different ways of interpreting this core idea, in particular different ways of understanding control. Segall cashes out 'control' (or rather responsibility) in terms of 'outcomes that would be unreasonable to expect the agent to avoid' (Segall 2010: 13). Thus, if an agent cannot be reasonably expected to avoid a certain outcome, s/he cannot be held responsible for (all) the consequences of her choice. If we combine this with the central thought of luck egalitarianism, we arrive at the conclusion that any inequalities that arise from decisions that agents cannot be expected to avoid are unjust and ought to be redressed at the bar of justice.

What does this entail in terms of a right to health? First, let us note from the outset that we might expect a luck egalitarian theory of justice to find justifying a right to health challenging because the amount of a good that people are entitled to in such a theory can vary in relation to their responsibility; a luck egalitarian would, more generally, find it difficult to ground any welfare rights, that is, rights that specify an outcome to be achieved. Even those luck egalitarians who oppose equality of resources in favour of the welfare currency do not advocate equality of welfare as such but rather equal *opportunity* for welfare or equal *access* to advantage, for instance.

For the same reason, luck egalitarianism poses a particular challenge for people who consider health special since it can lead to the conclusion that people who gamble with their health are not owed anything if they lose the gamble. It is thus not unfair to deny treatment to people who contract lung cancer because of smoking, for example. This implication of luck egalitarianism has attracted a lot of criticism, in the form of the 'abandonment of the imprudent' objection, which presupposes that this result is counter-intuitive. For that reason, Segall, among others, wants to show that a luck egalitarian theory is consistent with a healthcare system that is universal, both in the sense of not excluding anyone and not allowing people to opt out. If such a healthcare system was shown to be a requirement of justice, it would yield a right to healthcare. However, Segall's argument ultimately fails to ground such a right.

What Segall argues in response to the abandonment objection is that the luck egalitarian can adopt a 'value pluralist' approach, according to which justice is only one among the values that should be realised in a society. So although the luck egalitarian account of justice does not *require* treating the imprudent, other values may imply that we have a duty to do so. He claims that the demands of fairness in this case are indeterminate; in other words, luck egalitarian justice neither requires nor prohibits treating the imprudent but does *allow* such treatment. If that is the case, we can – he further argues – supplement justice with other considerations, such as basic needs, in order to show that the luck egalitarian need not abandon the imprudent.

This argument is flawed in my view. Segall's assertion that luck egalitarianism allows treating the imprudent ignores one side of the luck egalitarian equation, namely the supply side, as it were. Segall claims that according to the luck egalitarian it is neither fair nor unfair to treat the imprudent. But while this may be the implication of a general statement of the luck egalitarian aim, other concerns of fairness may indicate that it is forbidden to treat the imprudent at the bar of justice. Let me explain. A standard statement of the luck egalitarian aim is that 'inequalities are unfair if and only if they are not due to people's choices'. Now this entails that we are required to correct those inequalities that are not due to choice and does not say anything about inequalities that *are* due to choice. In this sense, it might be read as allowing that the imprudent be treated. But in order to provide treatment to the lung cancer patient, the luck egalitarian must impose a duty to provide treatment and/or resources on others, who may not be liable for the costs incurred by the imprudent. Coercing people into covering costs that they are not responsible for goes against the luck egalitarian aim.[4] Furthermore, given the scarcity of such resources –

particularly labour power, when it comes to healthcare – this may mean denying treatment to other individuals who cannot be held responsible for their condition.

Nevertheless, I agree with Segall that luck egalitarianism does not forbid treating the imprudent, in the sense that it does not forbid *voluntary* transfers to the imprudent.[5] Thus luck egalitarianism does indeed allow treating the imprudent *voluntarily* and other requirements (of morality) may imply that treatment is in fact required. What follows is that we may have a duty to treat the imprudent but *not at the bar of justice.* If it is values *other than* justice that recommend treating the imprudent, this is not a duty of justice but rather a matter of charity or solidarity. In other words, the imprudent does not have a *right* to be treated. This need not be a problem for Segall, who does not seek to argue for such a right,[6] but I would maintain that his argument also fails to justify universal healthcare. A universal healthcare system relies on taxes, so allowing universal access to healthcare essentially means forcibly imposing the costs for the treatment of the imprudent on 'innocent' others. Segall ultimately resorts to a 'concern for meeting basic needs' in order to justify universal healthcare, which is the same strategy that human rights theorists adopt and which, I argued, is at best incomplete. So it seems that luck egalitarianism cannot ground a right to health or healthcare. In that case, is there anything that luck egalitarianism can and should recommend specifically in the area of health?

Perhaps the luck egalitarian can take a different route in order to argue for a right to health.[7] The luck egalitarian might apply the general argument from equal opportunity for welfare or equal access to advantage to the area of health and perhaps this is what a right to health is best understood as: a right to the conditions, including healthcare, that would enable one to lead a healthy life rather than a certain level of health. Note that this would no longer be a right to health *per se*, that is, to a certain health outcome, but rather an umbrella term for rights to other health-relevant goods.[8] This might seem like a straightforward argument but I will argue that it is a lot more problematic than it seems.

In order to justify equal opportunity for health one would have to be a luck egalitarian *specifically* about health and claim that it is unfair if someone is worse off in terms of health due to factors outside their control. This would mean that we would be required to neutralise the effects of luck on health, that is to say, it would require neutralising the effects of the social determinants of health and genetic factors.[9] But here the luck egalitarian encounters a bit of a dilemma. If our socio-economic status has an impact on our health but this status is the result of our voluntary choices, why neutralise its impact on health?

On the one hand, if the luck egalitarian claims that the resulting inequality in (opportunity for) health is unproblematic, no right to health can be argued for and a theory of justice *in health* appears redundant. If, on the other hand, the luck egalitarian wants to insist on equal opportunity for health, it seems that she must give up on a luck egalitarian distribution overall or more specifically on responsibility. One could claim that even if the distribution of health is the result of a fair distribution (of other goods), we need to neutralise the impact of factors beyond one's control on health. This seems to lead to a contradiction within luck egalitarianism since achieving luck egalitarian justice in one area seems to require upsetting that same requirement in another.

A possible way out of this conundrum would be to appeal to a more sophisticated view of responsibility whereby we might be able to claim that one cannot/should not be held responsible all the way down, as it were. In other words, we might be responsible for our socio-economic status but, inasmuch as this influences our decisions about health or our health *directly*, we should not be held (fully) responsible for our health status. The idea is that the decisions we make about our socio-economic status should not be taken as choices we make about every area of our lives. So luck egalitarians might be able to argue, in conjunction with the assumption that health is special, that we should ensure that our health status only depends on our decisions about health specifically and these should be fully voluntary, in the sense of being unconstrained by social or economic factors.

This would be a problematic and ambitious argument but let us assume that it works. The question is then whether it grounds a right to health, in the sense of equal opportunity for health. In order to answer this question, we need to know how we can neutralise the effects of factors beyond our control on health. And here we should distinguish between two levels at which we might intervene in order to improve the health status of individuals: we can prevent people getting ill or we can cure illnesses. So in order to neutralise the effects of social factors on health we can recommend eliminating their effect at the first level, that is, at the level of causing illness. But this means, on the one hand, that we might have to alter the otherwise just distribution of the social determinants of health. This is not only inconsistent, as I pointed out above, but it is also not sufficient to achieve equal opportunity for health, given the differential initial risks that people are exposed to. But there is a second route, namely neutralising the effect of factors outside our control by curing illness, that is, by providing healthcare! There will, of course, be cases when a cure is not available and for such cases the luck egalitarian can only recommend compensation.

So a luck egalitarian commitment to justice in health cannot generate an equal right to health *per se*, but it may be able to justify a principle of equal opportunity for health. Nevertheless, this translates into access to healthcare rather a right to health *per se*, although we should note that the argument does not necessarily entail a universal healthcare system. Some individuals may be excluded if they can be held responsible for their health status. Nevertheless, since luck egalitarianism requires neutralising the effects of brute luck, it arguably recommends unconditional treatment for all those conditions that are caused by brute luck and in that sense it may entail a right to healthcare.

Fair Equality of Opportunity

If a luck egalitarian theory does not yield a right to health we might look at a different egalitarian theory, in particular one that does not place much emphasis on personal responsibility, such as Daniels' account. The assumption that Daniels starts from, and that I share, is that 'the appeal to a right to health or to health care is not an appropriate starting point for an inquiry into just health or just health care' (Daniels 2008). 'Rather, we may claim a right to health or healthcare only if it can be harvested from an acceptable general theory of distributive justice or from a more particular theory of justice for health and health care' (Daniels 2008: 15).

Unlike Segall, Daniels explicitly talks about a (human) right to health and he denies that his account generates a right to health *per se*. He points out that 'health is an inappropriate object' of a right; 'if my poor health is not the result of anyone's doing, or failing to do, something for me or to me, that might have prevented or might cure my condition, then it is hard to see how any right of mine is being violated' (Daniels 2008: 145). Nevertheless, he claims that his argument supports both a right to health and healthcare. 'If we have an obligation to ensure fair equality of opportunity, we have an obligation to promote normal functioning, and our moral right to health and health care is the corollary of these obligations' (Daniels 2008: 316). He maintains, however, that the right to health should not be understood as a right to certain health outcomes but rather as a claim that 'certain individuals or groups or society as a whole must perform various actions, such as designing certain institutions and distributing important goods in certain ways, that promote or maintain or restore their health and must refrain from actions that interfere with it' (Daniels 2008: 145). In other words, the right to health becomes what I referred to above as an umbrella term for a cluster of rights to health-relevant goods. I submit, however, although I will not defend this position here, that this is not a right to health since it is reducible to rights other than health; furthermore, nothing is gained in my view by subsuming all of them under the banner of health.

So I want to see whether his account generates a principle of equality in health or universal healthcare since I started from the assumption that this is how rights to health can be justified. However, I want to argue that his theory is even less congenial to a right to healthcare and that the only right that emerges from it is a right to a sufficient level of health, which is a right to a specific health outcome.

In his previous book, *Just Health Care*, Daniels argued for universal healthcare, on the assumption that healthcare is a necessary (and sufficient) ingredient of good health. Given the recent empirical findings which show that some of the 'determinants' of health are social factors, Daniels has broadened his argument, while preserving the link between fair equality of opportunity and health. Daniels' general argument, in a nutshell, runs as follows: 1) health (understood as normal functioning) helps to protect opportunity and 2) justice as fairness requires protecting opportunity so justice as fairness requires protecting health and therefore meeting health needs (Daniels 2008: 30). The first premise as well as the validity of this argument is open to question but a thorough discussion of it is beyond the scope of this chapter; my aim is to see what kind of rights this argument might generate.

We might expect that, if it is the case that health promotes opportunity and equality of opportunity is a requirement of justice, this account leads to equality in health. But Daniels does not want to claim that inequality in health status is unjust. This is because not all inequality in health undermines fair equality of opportunity; not all shortfalls in health necessarily undermine access to opportunity and health should be understood as 'normal functioning' for the purposes of this argument. So it is only when people fall below the level of normal functioning that equality of opportunity is undermined. But perhaps Daniels could still maintain that health inequalities are unjust if, for instance, they are due to socially controllable factors regardless of the connection between health and opportunity. Daniels denies that a health inequality is unjust unless 'it results from an unjust distribution of the socially controllable determinants of population health' (Daniels 2008: 140). So a concern with equal opportunity and therefore health does not yield equality in health and right to health but only a claim to a fair distribution of the social determinants of health, that is, rights other than health. As pointed out above, this is not a genuine right to health.

But since healthcare might be part of this package of health-related goods, perhaps Daniels' argument could support a right to healthcare, in the sense of universal access to healthcare, which is indeed what he was arguing for in *Just Health Care*. Since he does not reject but only seeks to broaden that argument in light of the findings on the social determinants of health, it is worth considering it.

However, Gopal Sreenivasan argues that the equal opportunity argument fails to support *universal* healthcare. The argument from equal opportunity has, according to him, two main steps: the first is that anyone who suffers a loss of health suffers a violation of her fair share of opportunity, and the second is that everyone entitled to a fair share of health is entitled to a fair share of healthcare. Both these steps, Sreenivasan argues, are invalid; the second one, as we have seen, is rendered untrue by the findings about the social determinants of health so, if what we are interested in is health, providing universal healthcare will be insufficient. But perhaps healthcare is still necessary; as we have seen in the previous section, providing healthcare is one way of correcting the impact of social factors on health. Indeed, if the first is valid, people who suffer a shortfall in health will still require healthcare if their fair share of opportunity is to be restored.

But we have seen that the first step is also invalid, that is, it is not the case that *any* loss of health diminishes one's fair share of opportunity. What Daniels argues is that any loss of health that impairs 'normal functioning' is detrimental to opportunity, where opportunity is to be interpreted as a 'normal range of opportunity' rather as a relative notion, as Sreenivasan claims. Thus, loss of normal functioning impairs access to the range of opportunities that everyone should have in a just society.[10] In other words, there seems to be a sufficientarian threshold when it comes to health, in Daniels' account. This seems to entail that access to healthcare is required at the bar of justice. But note that this does not justify *universal* and unconditional access to healthcare. It only requires access to healthcare inasmuch as this is required to restore normal functioning. If there are conditions that do not impair normal functioning or, indeed, impairment of functioning that does not affect access to opportunities, like in the case of the elderly (Segall 2010: 32), it is not unjust to withhold healthcare. So this argument does not ground a right to healthcare, especially since it does not necessarily require treatment for conditions due to one's genetic make-up.

Nevertheless, this argument can in fact ground a right to a *sufficient* level of health or perhaps health *per se*, if health is by definition just normal functioning. So, in spite of Daniels' denial that health is an appropriate subject of a right, it seems that his argument from fair equality of opportunity, if successful, yields an equal right to certain health outcomes, which may translate in unequal access to healthcare.

So neither of the two egalitarian theories that we considered can ground a right to the 'highest attainable level of health'. However, each of them claims to justify a more limited right to either healthcare or health. I argued that a luck egalitarian theory of justice in health could generate a (limited) right to healthcare, while a Rawlsian theory is more likely to insist on equality in terms of health outcomes, which could yield a right to the 'lowest level of health necessary', so to speak, rather than the highest attainable one.

The next question is then whether this could be a universal human right. I started from the assumption that if a theory of distributive justice can generate a right to health, this could in principle be a universal human right, unless there are further constraints that restrict the application of a theory to the domestic level. Indeed, Daniels explicitly rejects the global scope of his account while Segall claims that his arguments apply not only globally but perhaps cosmically. But even if these theories could be applied globally, there are some specific challenges that are posed by the concept of human rights, which I will consider in the next section.

POSITIVE RIGHTS AND (IM)PERFECT DUTIES

In this last section, I will briefly examine an argument put forward by Onora O'Neill, according to which positive rights cannot be human rights because the duties they entail are not clearly specified and, if institutions are appealed to in order to specify these duties, they become special rather than general rights. This point, as she presents it, is meant to be a merely conceptual point rather than a normative one. What I want to argue is that this conclusion does not follow as a matter of conceptual truth but it is rather based on normative assumptions. The implications of my argument are quite modest; I do not claim to have shown that there is a human right to health or indeed any other positive rights. The argument only shows, against O'Neill, that not all positive rights are ineligible as pre-institutional, general rights; however, if some positive rights are to be human rights, their correlative duties must be clearly specified and this seems to imply that rights to a certain amount of goods, such as healthcare, are more plausible candidates.

O'Neill shares the assumptions about human rights outlined at the start of this chapter. More specifically, she assumes that moral human rights must be general rather than special, thus pre-institutional, which means that the duties correlative to them must be pre-institutional as well. Her argument is thus directed at the welfare or socio-economic rights currently enshrined in international law. A terminological clarification may be in order here. O'Neill finds the language of 'welfare' rights inaccurate since this expression simply refers, in her view, to rights to goods and services rather than rights that serve the welfare of the recipient. I agree with this point, but at the same time, positive rights can be expressed, as I suggested throughout, either as entitlements to a certain outcome or as claims to goods and services, regardless of the outcome to be achieved. I reserve the term 'welfare rights' for the former.

First, O'Neill argues against the view of human rights as 'aspirational', which is common among critics and supporters alike. Many positive human rights, including the right to health, are seen as ideals to be realised 'progressively', to the extent that states can afford their realisation. But this view fails to ascribe human rights any normative force; if they are to be taken seriously as normative claims, their correlative duties must be taken seriously as well. But the duties correlative to human rights in international law are ascribed to states. This, as O'Neill correctly points out, would make them special rather than general rights. The question is then whether it is *possible* to see socio-economic rights as general rights. O'Neill suggests a negative answer, since in her view perfect universal obligations can only correspond to liberty rights (O'Neill 1996: 152). Her argument seems to run as follows:

1. all rights (including positive rights) have correlative obligations
2. duties correlative to rights must be perfect
    positive duties cannot be perfect unless they are special
3. Therefore, positive rights cannot have (general) correlative duties.

In the next few paragraphs I want to challenge the last assumption, but in order to do that we should look at the previous one as well. O'Neill concedes – to libertarians – that there is a significant difference between negative, 'liberty' rights and positive rights to goods and services. When it comes to negative or liberty rights, it is clear that all others have the same duty and there is no doubt who violates a right. But when it comes to rights to goods and services, 'there is systematic unclarity about whether one can speak of violators' (O'Neill 1996: 132). The assumption here is that these rights do not and cannot have specified correlative obligations.

It is often replied, as O'Neill remarks, that corresponding obligations could be assigned to specific agents; thus a positive right would correlate with a 'distributed obligation' that falls on specified agents or institutions. But O'Neill correctly points out that this would mean that positive rights are special rather than universal human rights. For these reasons, she concludes that the only genuine human rights are negative ones and if we are to be concerned with people's needs or well-being we must go beyond the framework of rights and pay closer attention to duties and virtues.

It seems to me that, while O'Neill's points are entirely justified, her conclusion is unwarranted. And that is because her assumption that positive duties cannot be general does not withstand scrutiny. This assumption is in turn based on the thought that duties correlative to rights must be perfect. But what exactly are perfect duties? There are several ways in which this requirement can be interpreted and I cannot discuss this in detail here, but let us accept that they must have a clearly specified content; more specifically, in my view, their content must be an *action* that is directed toward the recipient of the duty. Imperfect duties by contrast make reference to a goal that must be achieved without, however, specifying ways to achieve it or what the limits are.[11]

In order to comply with imperfect duties, agents must (continuously) strive to achieve the goal.

O'Neill presents the assumption that correlative duties must be perfect as a requirement that simply follows from the concept of a right, and that is to an extent true but it is a normative rather than a conceptual requirement. All rights, we established, must have correlative duties. But there is in principle no reason why such correlative duties cannot be imperfect, in the sense just outlined. Thus, it is conceptually possible that my right to be well-fed, for instance, correlates with your duty to do your best to feed me. This does not necessarily indicate a particular action that should be taken but it implies that the duty is only discharged when the goal, that is, being well-fed, is achieved.

A further assumption, however, is that rights are by definition enforceable claims; this is to say that it is permissible (for the right-holder or someone else) to force the bearer of the corresponding duty to discharge his/her obligations. It is, I believe, this assumption that motivates the claim that correlative duties must be perfect. Enforcing obligations that are not clearly specified or specified in terms of a goal – perhaps an ambitious one – to be achieved may be illegitimate, not in the least because it would be overly demanding; this is, however, a normative point. And what follows from this is that *welfare* rights, that is, rights to a state of affairs specified in terms of an outcome, are not enforceable hence not genuine rights but not that positive rights cannot be general.

So genuine rights must indeed correlate with perfect duties. Can duties to provide goods and services be perfect? O'Neill would have us believe that positive duties can only be perfect if they are special. But there seems to be no reason why a right to a good or a service cannot be held against all others, who would therefore have a duty of justice to provide the right-holder with the good or the service in question. Again, a further implicit assumption here is that not every person can have a duty to provide the *whole* good or service to each other person. Thus, they must be provided to one person by all others *collectively*. If that is the case, the obligation must be distributed so that each duty-bearer must provide a share of the good.

But this does not show that each other person has no perfect duty to provide this share and there is no reason why institutions are necessary in order to assign shares. What is, however, necessary is that the right itself is specified in terms of a *fixed* amount of a good or service that is divisible among all potential duty-bearers. This may be more easily achieved for rights to certain goods but it is not impossible for services. The unclarity then about who the rights-violators are in particular cases need not be as 'systematic' as O'Neill claims. If a right is unfulfilled, it will be possible to identify a rights violator once shares have been assigned. So it seems that the thought that positive rights cannot be general is insufficiently supported, to say the least. This suggests that a right to healthcare rather than health is more plausible as a human right.

CONCLUSION

I argued in this chapter that a human right to 'the highest attainable level of health' is not a genuine human right and I suggest that nothing is gained by positing such a right. In order to see whether a more modest right can be justified, I examined two theories of justice in health and concluded that neither of them can generate a right to health as such but can perhaps yield a right to healthcare or to a minimum/sufficient amount of health.

Part of the aim of this chapter, however, was also to motivate the view that in justifying certain (human) rights, both the rights-based and the distributive justice approach are insufficient. Instead we should approach the issue from both ends in order to see what rights can be matched with perfect universal obligations. This is the kind of analysis that I tried to undertake here and I tentatively concluded that a right to healthcare, and perhaps a certain amount of healthcare, is more plausible as a universal human right.

Notes

1. I am grateful to Anca Gheaus, Patti Tamara Lenard, Shlomi Segall, Christine Straehle and Kristin Voigt for their very helpful comments on a previous draft of this chapter.
2. For the distinction between general and special rights, see H. L. Hart 1984: 87–8.
3. By this I mean that a theory of justice should yield a just set of *moral* rights that in turn would underwrite a just legal system.
4. It could be argued that taxing those who also made risky choices but were lucky is legitimate. But this is actually a different argument. It challenges the notions of luck and responsibility employed and it seems to imply that

treating the *unlucky* imprudent is *required* rather than merely allowed. In any case, it is not Segall's argument.

5. For an argument to the contrary, see Kristin Voigt (2007), who argues that luck egalitarianism even forbids such transfers. This is, I take it, plausible only if the luck egalitarian principle is treated as an over-arching principle of morality, rather than as a narrow principle of distributive justice. I subscribe to the latter view.

6. Although he does not want to argue against a right to health or rights in general either. Personal communication.

7. I now depart from Segall's account and I try to construct a possible luck egalitarian argument for justice in health.

8. It seems like many interpretations of the legal duties that follow from the right to health actually envisage this kind of view, in spite of the wording of article 12 of ICESCR.

9. Many discussions of the social determinants of health proceed as though some of these factors are the *sole causes* of ill-health, which is far from clear. But I leave this otherwise very important complication aside here.

10. For other criticisms of Daniels' argument, and especially the notion of 'normal opportunity range', see Allen Buchanan 1984: 62–6.

11. O'Neill offers three different interpretations of what imperfect duties could be understood as but reasons of space prevent from examining them (O'Neill 1989: 224–5).

Chapter 2

WHAT'S WRONG WITH GLOBAL HEALTH INEQUALITIES?[1]

Daniel M. Hausman

Over the past century, there have been striking improvements in health across the earth, including among many of its poorest and initially least healthy people. In India and China, which together include more than one-third of the world's population, life expectancy has increased by more than twenty-five years since 1950. In China, life expectancy now stands at seventy-three years and trails that in Europe by only about three years. Those concerned about health have a great deal to celebrate.

The celebration is, however, spoiled by the glaring exceptions, which are clustered in sub-Saharan Africa, where life expectancies are typically in the forties and fifties. Hundreds of millions of individuals will have decades less of life than those who made better choices about where to be born, and their shorter lives will be burdened with more illnesses and disabilities. According to the *World Health Report 2000*, disability-adjusted life expectancy in Sierra Leone is under twenty-six!

Unlike the mass death and suffering caused by the 2010 earthquake in Haiti or the 2004 Indian Ocean tsunami, these global health inequalities seem to me, as to many others, not just a tragedy but also a moral outrage. What distinguishes the world's massive health inequalities from natural disasters is that the inequalities are up to us and consequently, unlike nature, subject to moral judgement. The forces of nature may do catastrophic harm, but they cannot do *wrong*. They are incapable of evil. The moral indignation that I and others experience when we think about global health inequalities pre-supposes that people can be blamed for these inequalities because there are feasible ways in which these inequalities could be eliminated or drastically mitigated.

This pre-supposition is justified. Though some of the excess mortality and disability in sub-Saharan Africa is due to a climate and geography in which infectious diseases thrive, climate and geography cannot be anything like the whole story. For example, Togo, Benin and Nigeria are located next to each other along the Gulf of Guinea. Their climates are similar, yet life expectancies are respectively 58, 57 and 47.[2] Nor can one explain health inequalities by adding in the effect of income inequalities, which, though due to human actions, are especially hard to address. The per capita GDPs of Togo ($858), Benin ($1,451) and Nigeria ($2,422) (IMF 2010)[3] would predict better rather than worse health in Nigeria. Although health inequalities have some connection to geography and poverty, they are not attributable solely to inequalities in income coupled with the unequal beneficence of nature.

Global health inequalities are morally bad, if for no reason other than the enormous and avoidable suffering and loss they involve. But does the problem lie specifically with the *inequalities*? Why should health any more than housing, diet or education be the same in different countries? And if the problem lies with the inequalities, does it lie with the inequalities specifically in health, or with more general inequalities in freedom, life prospects or well-being? In addition, is there anything special about health inequalities among countries, or should we be no less or no more concerned about health inequalities within countries?

We do not live in a world where health in the worst-off countries or regions is bad merely in comparison with health in more fortunate regions. In the world as we find it, those with appreciably worse health have bad health, a low level of well-being and very limited opportunities. Under-five mortality in Haiti is not only more than twice that in the Dominican Republic (with which it shares the island of Hispaniola), but it is almost one in fourteen. So there will be few practical differences between those who are concerned with inequalities specifically in health and those who are concerned with inequalities in opportunity or well-being. Nor will there be large practical differences between either of these egalitarians and benevolent non-egalitarians who are concerned about poor health, low well-being or limited opportunities. In some regards, this is fortunate, because it means that action to address global health inequalities does not need to wait for philosophical consensus on what exactly is wrong with them. But there remain important questions to be asked about the moral significance of health differences across nations, regions and ethnic groupings. It is these questions with which I shall be concerned.

Current global inequalities in overall health seem to me (as to many others) obviously unjust. In many cases, they result from horrendous rights violations, and they are correlated with unjust inequalities in well-being or opportunity. But apart from their causes, consequences and correlates, is there something unjust about health inequalities themselves?

In my 2007 essay, 'What's Wrong with Health Inequalities?', I argued that the answer is 'No'. I maintained that apart from one important exception, health inequalities among individuals are not in themselves injustices and that they do not imply the inequalities that raise questions of justice. Though I still defend this view, it is largely orthogonal to questions concerning inequalities in health across nations. International inequalities consist of inequalities in group averages, not in inequalities across individuals. They say nothing about how health is distributed within countries and only place a lower bound on the extent of health inequality across individuals. In comparing health in different countries (as measured by, for example, quality or disability-adjusted life years), one is unavoidably examining correlations between health and citizenship or residency, rather than considering the distribution of health across individuals. So questions about whether it is best to focus on the distribution of health itself or the way in which health correlates with other factors are moot.

My philosophical inquiry is organised as follows. Section 1 asks, 'What is wrong with inequality?' and focuses on the answer that so-called 'luck egalitarians' offer. Section 2 considers whether there are moral objections to inequalities specifically in health. Section 3 presents an alternative to the luck egalitarian view of the significance of inequalities and considers how this alternative applies to global inequalities. Section 4 comments on Norman Daniels' influential views, and Section 5 concludes.

1. WHAT IS WRONG WITH INEQUALITY?

What mainly motivates global egalitarians are the huge disparities in life prospects between those who grow up in affluent and secure circumstances and those who grow up in extreme poverty or in abusive, chaotic circumstances. Most people feel that inequalities like these are seriously unjust. One explanation for these intuitions is that morality includes a fundamental egalitarian principle to the effect that:

(1) Other things being equal, inequalities are unjust.

The 'other things being equal' clause is crucial, because equality is not the only relevant consideration. Larger inequalities accompanied by greater welfare may be better than greater equality with lower welfare.

(1) is as stated indefensible. Only some differences among people, such as the differences in opportunity or well-being implicit in a twenty-year difference in life expectancy, are of moral concern. Small inequalities in well-being or specific inequalities in things such as numbers of rings or piercings are not of moral concern. Furthermore, as I have already argued, egalitarians need not object to inequalities that cannot be remedied by human action. So a fundamental egalitarian principle might instead be formulated as:

(2) Other things being equal, significant inequalities in overall well-being that could be addressed by human action or social institutions are unjust.

Most contemporary egalitarians would maintain that there is nothing unjust about some inequalities, such as those that obtain between innocent citizens and convicted thieves.[4] It is open to an egalitarian to object to inequalities regardless of any questions about responsibility or desert and to explain our intuition that the thief ought to be worse off in terms of competing non-egalitarian moral considerations such as retribution or desert. But most egalitarians have instead felt that there is no moral reason at all to favour equality when those who are worse off are responsible for their plight. Through this line of thought, one arrives at a vague 'luck egalitarian' sufficient condition for injustice:

(3) Other things being equal, significant inequalities in overall well-being for which individuals are not responsible that could be addressed by human action or social institutions are unjust.

Kok-Chor Tan states what he takes to be the core of luck egalitarianism as '[P]ersons should not be disadvantaged or advantaged simply on account of bad or good luck' (Tan 2008: 665). (3) provides only a vague sufficient condition (other things being equal) for injustice. But in the context of international health inequalities, this sufficient condition is very important, for what could be more a matter of brute luck than the country one happens to be born in? This sufficient condition does not say that, other things being equal, inequalities for which individuals are responsible are just. It thus falls short of defining how inequalities matter to justice. If one were to treat the condition in (3) as both necessary and sufficient, one might formulate egalitarianism as:

(4) Other things being equal, significant inequalities in overall well-being that could be addressed by human action or social institutions are unjust if and only if individuals are not responsible for them.

There appear, however, to be serious objections to the necessary condition implied by (4). I shall mention three. The first, which is due to Elizabeth Anderson (1999), is the problem of 'the abandonment of the imprudent'. For example, suppose that through imprudent choices in her early twenties, for which Ann is fully responsible, she finds herself at age thirty with few skills, a criminal record, disabilities and no one to care for her. Ann's society offers her no assistance. According to (4) there are no egalitarian objections to Ann's harsh society.

Second, consider the case of Amy who is badly off because she has contracted a contagious disease in the course of heroically tending to others. Her society, like Ann's, does nothing for her, because she is responsible for her own bad health. (4) implies that an egalitarian has no grounds upon which to criticise abandoning the self-sacrificing.

Luck egalitarians can respond to these objections either by accepting the verdict that there are no egalitarian objections to Ann's or Amy's societies and emphasising other, non-egalitarian, objections or, like Tan (2008) and Shlomi Segall (2010), maintaining that there are other egalitarian considerations, such as a requirement that everyone's basic needs be met, which are not satisfied by societies such as Ann's or Amy's. On the latter view, luck-egalitarian concerns are not the whole of an egalitarian account of justice.

A third objection to (4) is that it favours 'levelling-down.' For example, it is possible to lower current health and well-being to levels typical of the world before the twentieth century. Assume that this loss in health and well-being has no benefits at all either now or in the future for anybody. Yet, if, as (4) maintains, all inequalities for which individuals are not responsible are objectionable, then there is an egalitarian reason in favour of making today's population worse off, even if, all things considered, it is morally impermissible. Those who make this objection regard this as an absurd implication. How could there be anything good about causing so much harm without benefit to anyone?

I believe that this objection confuses the moral assessment of the distribution of well-being before and after making people worse off with the moral assessment of harming people. Luck egalitarians should condemn the latter because making people worse off fails to show respect to individuals whose well-being is sacrificed. But that does not imply that the resulting distribution cannot be better from an egalitarian perspective. So I do not think that the levelling-down objection has much to it.

But the abandonment of the imprudent and of the self-sacrificing show that there are injustices other than inequalities for which individuals are not responsible. So let us retreat to (3) and concede that it only captures a portion of what the egalitarian demands.

The notion of responsibility mentioned in (3) is problematic. According to Richard Arneson, people are responsible for 'the foreseeable consequences of their voluntary choices' (Arneson 1989: 88). Causal responsibility and hence, as G. A. Cohen (1989) insists, free will are necessary for the relevant sort of responsibility, but not sufficient. Until it became known that smoking causes lung cancer, smokers bore no responsibility in the relevant sense for contracting lung cancer, even if they freely chose to smoke. By linking responsibility to free will, Cohen and Arneson tie the conclusions of egalitarianism to metaphysical inquiries concerning free will, which do not appear to have much to do with the intuitive distinctions people make between inequalities that are unjust and inequalities that are just. Ronald Dworkin, in contrast, does not require free will for responsibility. In his view, individuals should be held responsible for actions that stem from 'those beliefs and attitudes that define what a successful life would be like, which the ideal assigns to the person', not for actions that are caused by 'those features of body or mind or personality that provide means or impediments to that success, which the ideal assigns to the person's circumstances' (Dworkin 1981: 303). But this is vague, and it is arguable that, in contrast to what Dworkin's view implies, people are responsible for the consequences of some psychological impediments to the pursuit of their objectives, such as compulsions or whims.

In contrast both to Cohen and Arneson and to Dworkin, Segall holds that an individual is not responsible for an outcome if it would have been unreasonable for society to expect the individual to avoid it. Segall's account is attractive as a sufficient condition on responsibility, but as a necessary condition it is implausible. An individual may be responsible for an action and its consequences, even though it is not reasonable to expect the individual to avoid the action. For example, it is not reasonable for society to expect a Jehovah's Witness to accept a blood transfusion, but Jehovah's Witnesses are in the relevant sense responsible for refusing to accept a transfusion and for the consequences that follow. A benevolent luck egalitarian would be saddened by the death of a Jehovah's Witness owing to his or her refusal to accept a transfusion, but the luck egalitarian would not see any injustice.

As the last two paragraphs show, it is not easy to provide an adequate account of responsibility. At the same time, one must be precise about what people are responsible for, if one is to judge whether inequalities are unjust. These issues are important in the context of global health inequalities. For example, are people responsible for those inequalities in health and well-being that depend on cultural differences? Individuals do not voluntarily choose their cultures, but they have some power to change their allegiances. A luck egalitarian who endorses an account of responsibility like Dworkin's or Segall's would find nothing objectionable in global inequalities that are due to cultural differences, unless those cultural differences were themselves the result of injustices. On the other hand, luck egalitarians might maintain that inequalities due to culture are unjust, on the grounds that people do not choose their culture.

Moreover, responsibility is usually shared: outcomes are almost always due both to individual choice and to circumstances over which individuals have no control. Those who smoke increase their risk of lung cancer, but they are still unlikely to get cancer. If smokers are responsible for their smoking (which is already questionable), how much responsibility should they bear for the inequalities due to bad outcomes that smoking makes somewhat more probable?

This section began with the intuition that the gross inequalities we observe in the world today constitute serious moral wrongs. One way to explain this intuition is to invoke some egalitarian principle to the effect that inequalities in the distribution of benefits and harms are morally objectionable. Other intuitions concerning responsibility pushed us toward a version of luck egalitarianism. But luck egalitarianism faces counter-examples, falls short of a comprehensive account of egalitarianism and seems not to capture some central egalitarian intuitions.

Is there no other way to understand what is wrong with current inequalities? One possibility is that what is wrong with these inequalities is simply the suffering and misery of those who are doing badly.[5] The importance specifically of the inequality lies in its demonstration that the suffering and misery of those doing badly is avoidable and hence a moral wrong. On this view, there is nothing intrinsically unjust or morally wrong about inequalities themselves; though the actual inequalities we observe, which involve great deprivation, constitute serious wrongs.

Another possibility, which I defend elsewhere (Hausman and Waldren 2011), is that egalitarianism is actually a family of related positions, with different egalitarians focusing on the distribution of different goods and with different reasons explaining why they take the distribution of these goods to be of moral importance (see also O'Neill 2008). So, for example, some egalitarians are concerned about the distribution of benefits and burdens by societies and especially by the state as the agent of society. A commitment to fairness and a particular construal of impartiality explains why egalitarians of this sort are so concerned with the distribution of benefits and burdens. (These egalitarians would not be as concerned about inequalities among different nations.) Other egalitarians are concerned about the distribution of status, power and respect, because they think that morality rests on equality of respect and moral standing and that relations among people should be governed by reciprocity. Still other egalitarians are motivated by a concern with solidarity and fraternity, and for that reason condemn large inequalities in wealth, status and power. What makes those concerned with solidarity, like those concerned with reciprocity, equality of respect or impartiality, all egalitarians is the fact that patterns of distribution constitute not merely cause, but the realisation or frustration of these ideals.

From this perspective, luck egalitarianism appears to be *superficial* as well as problematic. Luck egalitarianism stipulates a concern with significant inequalities in welfare or opportunities without providing philosophical foundations for this concern. It never explains *why* distributive inequality matters.[6] Both to justify luck egalitarianism and to explain how it should cope with the difficulties canvassed above, much more needs to be said about its moral foundations. The only author I know of who has sketched a foundation for luck egalitarianism is Larry Temkin, who grounds his version of luck egalitarianism in considerations of desert.[7] His view condemns both undeserved inequalities and undeserved *equalities*, because rewards should match deserts. The emphasis on desert nicely explains the intuition that the imprudent should neither be fully compensated nor abandoned altogether, while those who have been disadvantaged as a result of admirable self-sacrifice should be compensated. The principle that people should get what they deserve is not, however, itself an egalitarian principle. With the additional assumption that there is a baseline equality of desert or that equality is the default when desert is not defined, Temkin's position is nevertheless arguably egalitarian. But since, unlike Temkin, most luck egalitarians do not ground their views in notions of desert, we are left where we were – with a doctrine lacking any support apart from providing one among several competing explanations for our outrage at the enormous inequalities that characterise the contemporary world.

2. EQUALITY OF HEALTH

Luck egalitarians want to eliminate differences in opportunities or welfare for which individuals are not responsible. Health strongly influences opportunity and welfare, and people are not responsible for much of their health. So the distribution of health will be of concern to luck egalitarians. But why should luck egalitarians want to equalise health outcomes for which individuals are not responsible?

To address this question in general, something should be said about what is meant by equality in health. In the context of international comparisons, we can take a shortcut. Provided that one can generate some snapshot summary measure of population health that is sensitive to both mortality and morbidity – which is far from an innocuous proviso (Hausman unpublished) – one can take the average health of members of two of the world's nations as equal if the summary measures of the health of those two populations are equal. A luck egalitarian would object to inequalities in average population health across countries, except insofar as members of different populations are responsible for the differences in their health. Clearly a luck egalitarian would also be concerned about inequalities within countries, but this essay is only concerned with inequalities across countries.

Let us then return to the question of what reason luck egalitarians might have to seek equality in average health across countries. For example, life expectancy in Paraguay for men is 69.7, while in Russia it is 59.3.[8] If one rules out levelling down, the only way to equalise health is to assist Russia to improve its health. But it could be that assisting Russia would amplify rather than mitigate the inequality in overall well-being. Per capita income in Russia is $10,437, more than three times the per capita income of $2,886 in Paraguay. Russia also scores higher in terms of the human development index (.719 compared to Paraguay's .640). Even if the assistance provided to Russia is narrowly focused on health, it is likely to increase the overall inequalities in welfare or opportunity. In a case such as this one, it would seem that a luck egalitarian should oppose equalising health. To mitigate the overall inequality in average well-being, Paraguay rather than Russia needs the additional resources.

Consider then a comparison like that between Estonia and Peru. Health, as indicated by both life expectancy and disability-adjusted life expectancy, is just about the same. Per capita income, however, is more than three times as large in Estonia ($14,238) as in Peru ($4,469). The human development index number for Estonia is also a good deal higher. Egalitarians will obviously not be content, even though health is equal. But what weight should equality of health have? In attempting to lessen the overall inequalities, should one aim to preserve the equality of health, or would it be better to compensate for the huge inequalities in income by improving health in Peru? Is there anything better about separately equalising both income and health, as opposed to equalising the situation by compensating inequalities in income and health? As far as I can see, nothing in luck egalitarianism in general favours equalising health.

There is, however, one special case where luck egalitarianism does favour specifically targeting health inequalities. To describe that case, some distinctions are needed (Hausman 2007). Some health deficiencies are preventable or curable – call these 'remediable' – while others are not. Some health deficiencies are compensable – individuals can be made just as well off by providing them with more of other resources – while others are incompensable. For example, a diabetic coma is incompensable, but remediable. Congenital blindness is irremediable but compensable. Tay Sachs disease is neither remediable nor compensable. Mild myopia is both remediable and compensable. Only serious health conditions will be incompensable.

Consider then a case in which Abby is better off than Zack because he has a remediable and incompensable health deficiency that Abby does not have. If Zack is not responsible for his health problem, then the luck egalitarian finds this state of affairs unjust. Since Zack's health problem is incompensable, the unjust inequality in well-being can only be addressed by eliminating the inequality in health. When health problems are remediable and incompensable and individuals are not responsible for them, then equalising opportunity for welfare will often require equalising health. Though this is a special case, it is at the core of the huge health disparities between the countries of sub-Saharan Africa and most of the rest of the world, which are due to remediable but serious and often fatal diseases. There is a strong egalitarian case to be made for specifically attacking those diseases.

3. RELATIONAL EGALITARIANISM AND HEALTH INEQUALITIES

As I mentioned briefly near the end of Section 1, I believe egalitarianism is a family of positions motivated by several distinct moral commitments that are egalitarian in their spirit, rationale and implications. The alternative to luck egalitarianism that has been most discussed in the literature focuses on equality of standing, respect and political power, because it sees equality as a matter of how individuals relate to one another. This relational egalitarianism, versions of which one finds in the work of Rawls (1971), Daniels (1985, 2007), Anderson (1999), Scheffler (2003a, 2005) and Freeman (2007), is grounded in a moral commitment to equal respect and a political commitment to reciprocity and liberty in the sense of non-domination. It is not mainly concerned with the distribution of benefits and burdens by state or society or with holdings of goods, except insofar as these impinge on the relations among individuals and threaten to subordinate some to others or to diminish the liberties of some relative to the liberties of others.

Many have taken relational egalitarianism to be irrelevant to inequalities among nations and as concerned exclusively with the relations among fellow citizens or residents of some political unit. But a concern with equal respect and non-domination and the ideal of reciprocity also ground concerns with the relations among individuals who share no bonds of citizenship or proximity.

A relational egalitarian has in general an easier time defending policies that mitigate health inequalities than does a luck egalitarian. Though in my view a relational egalitarian cannot make a case for strict equality of health, large inequalities in health undermine reciprocity and equal respect. Health inequalities within nations render individuals vulnerable to domination by others and limit their domestic political voice. Similarly, health inequalities across national boundaries render individuals in one nation vulnerable to domination by other nations and diminish their voice in international co-operation. The case for diminishing health inequalities then rests on the claim that significant inequalities in health, unlike inequalities in goods in general, are crucial to maintaining equality in status and the possibility of reciprocity. 'Status' is ambiguous. It refers both to civic status, which is a relation among citizens or residents of a single country, and to a more fundamental moral status, which is a relation among human beings, regardless of their citizenship. Although the effects of ill-health on well-being are often compensable, the effects on the political and social relations among individuals are not readily compensable, and there is consequently an egalitarian case to be made for mitigating health inequalities, even in circumstances in which there are inequalities in well-being that might be aggravated by the lessening of health inequalities. This relational egalitarian case is stronger with respect to inequalities within countries, and the limits it places on inequalities within countries are more stringent than the limits it places on inequalities among countries, but relational egalitarianism limits international as well as domestic inequalities.

At the same time that a relational egalitarian like me would condemn the outrageous inequalities in health and life prospects between so many of those who live in sub-Saharan Africa and most of the rest of the world's population, I doubt that the objective should be that the health of all nations (as measured in disability or quality-adjusted life years) should be just the same. Just as there is no injustice in the inequality between the life expectancy of individuals who take few risks and the life expectancy of rock-climbers, so there is no injustice if international health inequalities reflect cultural differences (which are not themselves the product of injustices). Many of the activities that people find fulfilling – whether they be matters of diet, recreation, child-rearing, ageing or social solidarity – bear on people's health; and though cultures evolve as knowledge of their consequences spreads, there is no ethical mandate for societies to maximise health without regard to other values.

4. DANIELS' VIEW

In his influential work on health and justice (1985, 2007), Norman Daniels rejects luck egalitarianism and draws on Rawl's relationally egalitarian *Theory of Justice*. Like Rawls, Daniels does not intend his account to apply to the assessment of health differences between different countries, and my discussion below thus extends Daniels' account. Daniels takes the distribution of health and healthcare to be governed by generalisations of Rawls' two principles of justice, and in particular by a generalisation of a portion of Rawls' second principle, which Rawls calls 'Fair Equality of Opportunity'. In Rawls' work (which abstracts from all health disparities), fair equality of opportunity obtains when people's social circumstances do not affect their career prospects. This principle diverges from luck egalitarianism, because it is not concerned with the distribution of overall well-being and because it permits career prospects (as well as well-being) to be influenced by an individual's talents and skills, even though individuals are typically not responsible for them.

Daniels points out that if one relaxes Rawls' simplification and allows for the possibility of ill-health, then one must recognise that societies can influence opportunity not only through social resources, but also via healthcare and public-health policies. Daniels here broadens the notion of opportunity. In his view, If P and Q have the same talents, then P has greater opportunities than Q if and only if P has access to a larger portion of the range of the life plans accessible to individuals with these talents than Q has. Comparing these ranges across nations rather than within a single country is a tricky business, because not all the same ways of living may exist in different countries. There are few Shamans in Canada or stock-traders in Tibet. But rough comparisons of the range of opportunities can still be made. Daniels is concerned to eliminate inequalities in opportunities for carrying out life plans that do not arise from differing talents.

Daniels is not a luck egalitarian, since he calls for no compensation for differences in talents, even though individuals are not responsible for those differences. But his view faces the same difficulties in justifying equalising health that the luck egalitarian faces. For example, despite having worse health than Paraguayans, Russians probably have access to a larger portion of the range of life plans open to modern-day people than do Paraguayans. Fair equality of opportunity (applied globally in this way) would not prioritise improving health in Russia. In addition, as argued above, one can equalise opportunities by compensating inequalities in health and social advantages or by separately equalising each. Nothing in Daniels' theory favours the latter (Sreenivasan 2007).

Moreover, in revising Rawls' fair equality of opportunity principle, Daniels undermines its egalitarian rationale. As Daniels emphasises, his version of the fair equality of opportunity principle requires prevention and treatment of disease or disability, not enhancement of non-pathological traits, even when these traits lead to overall functioning that significantly diminishes opportunity. Non-pathological traits – abilities and skills – define what someone's fair share of the normal opportunity range is, while pathological traits prevent individuals from enjoying their fair share. So on Daniels' view, someone whose short stature is due to a (pathological) growth-hormone deficiency should be treated with growth hormone while someone of equal stature without a hormone deficiency who is equally sensitive to growth hormone need not be treated (see Buchanan et al. 2000: 115).

What leads to this conclusion is Daniels' view that fair equality of opportunity requires mitigation of pathologies but tolerates inequalities due to differences in talents. This way of distinguishing the cases thus places enormous weight on the distinction between 'low talent' and pathology (Jacobs 1996: 337), which, according to the account of health that Daniels relies on, is in fact largely arbitrary.[9] In addition, what reason could a relational egalitarian have to favour remediation or compensation for conditions depending on whether they are due to pathologies or to talent deficiencies? Surely what matters is how a condition affects people and the possibilities and costs of remedy or compensation, not whether it counts as a disease.

The fact that Daniels' version of the fair equality of opportunity principle justifies the disparate treatment of conditions depending on whether they result from pathology or from low talent casts doubt on the principle. In Rawls' hands, the principle had a clear rationale from a relational egalitarian perspective. Allowing social factors such as one's family's wealth and status to influence opportunities for careers and positions fails to show equal respect and facilitates domination of some people by others, while allowing talents and motivation to influence opportunities for careers and positions need not do so. But relational egalitarians have no reason to be more concerned about inequalities due to poor health than about inequalities due to differences in talents. Daniels' version of fair equality of opportunity has no relational egalitarian rationale.

If Daniels were instead to regard inequalities in opportunities to achieve life plans due to talents as just as unacceptable as inequalities due to poor health, then his view would become a form of luck egalitarianism where the object of distributional concern consists in the range of accessible life plans rather than well-being. The resulting view would have much the same rationale as more standard variants of luck egalitarianism; and it would be no better able to justify equalising health.

5. JUSTIFYING THE MITIGATION OF HEALTH INEQUALITIES

Most luck egalitarians have been concerned about inequalities in overall well-being for which individuals are not responsible. Relational egalitarians have been concerned about differences in moral standing, political influence and the extent to which some individuals can dominate others. Other egalitarians have been more concerned about impartiality or solidarity. Apart from uncertainties about how to treat inequalities due to cultural differences, luck egalitarian approaches apply in the same way to inequalities across national boundaries as they do to inequalities within countries. Other versions of egalitarianism, in contrast, which emphasise impartiality of state action, solidarity and reciprocity, apply more directly and stringently to inequalities within countries. If international health inequalities are of egalitarian concern, it must be because of their bearing on inequalities in well-being for which individuals are not responsible, their implications for the relations among people, whether they conflict with the impartiality and fairness required of the state, or because of their bearing on solidarity. Since equalising health is not a necessary condition for achieving the goals of the luck egalitarian and indeed sometimes impedes those goals, luck egalitarians cannot justify the claim that health inequalities are *prima facie* unjust. Relational egalitarians, in contrast, can make a case against large health inequalities, especially within a single country, but not in the way Norman Daniels attempts to do so.

Are there no other grounds upon which to condemn health inequalities? In addition to a variety of not altogether convincing practical political considerations, I think that two arguments can be made. The strongest egalitarian criticisms of domestic inequalities in health rest, I think, on the values of solidarity and reciprocity, which, as I argued above, I take to be themselves egalitarian values. Just about everybody is sometimes sick and in need of aid, and collectively we are able (to varying extents) to protect, cure or comfort those who are stricken. By guaranteeing that we will assist one another in times of need, we recognise our common vulnerability and affirm our common humanity. The protection of life and basic functioning and the alleviation of physical and mental suffering have a special significance, since everything of value in human life depends on them. To permit some to suffer, to die or to be disabled needlessly is to fail to embrace them as partners in the human enterprise. This is, in rough outline, what I take to be the central egalitarian basis for condemning incompensable inequalities in health.

But the extent to which solidarity is possible across national boundaries is limited, and this argument has less application to international inequalities. The strongest reason to condemn international inequalities, I believe, turns out not to be an egalitarian reason: large international health inequalities in fact cause great suffering. Relatively small transfers of resources to the impoverished to improve nutrition and sanitation and to provide treatments for common diseases would diminish inequalities in health and at the same time increase total well-being both directly and through improvements in the labour force.[10] Though one can easily imagine circumstances in which inequalities in health would increase rather than decrease human suffering, those circumstances are not ours.

This last argument for the egalitarian conclusion that we should act to lessen inequalities in the distribution of health does not rest on any egalitarian premises, but it is none the worse for that. Indeed, given how contentious egalitarianism is, the possibility of making a non-egalitarian argument for diminishing inequalities in health and healthcare should be welcomed.

Notes

1. I am indebted to the editors and to J. Paul Kelleher for comments on an earlier draft of this essay.
2. From the United Nations list 2005–10. According to the *CIA World Fact Book*, the life expectancies are 59, 59 and 47 (Wikipedia 2011). According

to the 2000 *World Health Report*, the disability adjusted life expectancy of Benin was best at 42, followed by 40 for Togo and 38 for Nigeria.

3. These comparisons rely on purchasing power parity rather than exchange rates.

4. Indeed, some egalitarians, such as Larry Temkin (1993, 2003), would argue that it would be unjust if thieves were living well. But this view seems to reflect considerations of desert, which are orthogonal to egalitarian concerns about responsibility. What distinguishes the imprisoned thief from the successful one is desert, not necessarily responsibility. If a luck egalitarian believes that there is an egalitarian objection to be made to a state of affairs in which an extremely capable criminal is better off than an untalented but honest hard worker, then it seems that the luck egalitarian is concerned about desert as well as responsibility.

5. '. . . what makes us care about various inequalities is . . . the hunger of the hungry, the need of the needy, the suffering of the ill, and so on. The fact that they are worse-off in the relevant respect than their neighbours is relevant. But it is relevant not as an independent evil of inequality. Its relevance is in showing that their hunger is greater, their need more pressing, their suffering more hurtful, and therefore our concern for the hungry, the needy, the suffering, and not our concern for equality makes us give them the priority.' (Raz 1984: 240)

6. Ironically, Tan argues that what distinguishes luck egalitarianism is that it is a 'grounding principle' that answers the question, 'Why does distributive inequality matter?' (2008: 667) – that is, that it answers the question that I am accusing it of failing to answer. What then, in his view, is the answer? According to Tan, the luck egalitarian holds that 'persons should not be disadvantaged simply because of bad luck' because 'individuals can only be held responsible for outcomes that are due to their own choices' (2008: 667). But the uncontroversial premise concerning responsibility says nothing at all about how advantages or disadvantages for which individuals should not be held responsible should be distributed. Tan never tells us how the luck egalitarian answers the question, 'Why does distributive inequality matter?'

7. I am indebted to Matt Waldren for this reading of Temkin (which Temkin accepts). Segall explicitly rejects such a justification for luck egalitarianism (2010: 16–17), and argues that his concerns are completely independent of questions of desert. But he provides no alternative philosophical rationale for his qualified luck egalitarianism. The only consideration in its favour is its questionable ability to match our intuitions.

8. According to *The World Health Report 2000*, disability adjusted life expectancies for men in Paraguay and Russia were respectively 63 and 56.

9. Daniels adopts Christopher Boorse's view (1977, 1997), according to which health is the absence of disease or pathology. According to Boorse, there is a pathology in some part of an organism when the level of functioning or capacity to function is in the lower tail of the distribution of efficiency of part function. Exactly where to draw the line between low normal and pathological functioning is in Boorse's view arbitrary. There is nothing in theoretical medicine or biology that tells one whether the bottom 5 per cent or 1 per cent or .001 per cent of liver function among some reference class divides the pathological from the non-pathological. For a critique of this view, see Schwarz 2007.

10. One might question this claim on the grounds that improving the health of those who are worst off would lead to a population explosion that would diminish future total well-being. The tragic scenario suggested by this objection might come to pass. But the future is too uncertain to justify a certain present loss of well-being.

Chapter 3

ECOLOGICAL SUBJECTS, 'ETHICAL PLACE-MAKING' AND GLOBAL HEALTH EQUITY

Lisa Eckenwiler

In this essay I begin by asking what research on societal determinants of health suggests for the specific ideals we should aspire toward in addressing global health inequities. I consider a set of theories of justice that seems best-suited to attend to societal determinants of health and find them wanting given an impoverished conception of subjects. I suggest, first, a slight shift in focus away from individual selves and propose an ethic of 'implacement' or 'place-making' for persons (re) conceived as ecological subjects. In making this argument I draw on a not-so-novel epistemological framework, ecological thinking, and demonstrate its value for understanding and responding to global health inequities. Ecological thinking, indeed, suggests new ideas about the ethical norms that should guide work for global health equity. At the same time, it helps to shine light on the sources of responsibility. I will also argue that the grounding of responsibility for global health equity can be found not merely in shared humanity, compassion and participation in the processes that generate injustice, but also in our nature as ecological subjects, that is, interdependent beings who are in a profound sense constitutive of one another. The social connections between us – 'across distance' as they are often framed – are even tighter than most theorising about global justice acknowledges.

EQUALITY OF WHAT?

The existence of global health inequalities has been well documented; and evidence concerning the societal determinants of these inequalities continues to mount (Marmot 2007, 2008; Birn 2011). The question I want to explore is: what should we aim for in addressing injustice, that is, inequity in global health, in light of what is known about the social determinants of health? While many lines of argument can be invoked concerning global justice and health equity, I refer to a select set because of their strength in attending to the importance of social structures in shaping people's prospects and, also, their movement away from thinking strictly about the distribution of resources, or what people have, toward their capacities, or what they 'are able to do and to be' (Nussbaum 2006: 70). What I will call 'enabling' conceptions of justice aim at attending to the social and political conditions that support people's capacities for self-development and self-determination. Iris Marion Young's theory of justice as enablement calls for reform of the social and institutional structures that systematically constrain people's capacities for self-development and self-determination and threaten their prospects for equality (Young 2006). Young defines injustice in terms of domination and oppression, which operate through social norms, economic relations and structures, and the organisation of decision-making processes to systematically constrain possibilities for some while at the same time expanding and enriching them for others. Carol Gould's notion of justice as 'equal positive freedom' requires not only 'the absence of constraining conditions such as coercion and oppression' but also access to the means or conditions for 'self-transformation' and the 'development of capacities and the realisation of projects over time'. Justice, here too, is about 'the availability of *enabling* [my emphasis] conditions' for individuals (Gould 2009: 165–6). Finally, the capabilities approach of Martha Nussbaum and Amartya Sen, a minimalist, agent-centred, universalistic account of global justice, emphasises people's capacities to be and to do. As Nussbaum underscores, here people's 'active striving' and 'achievement' matter in assessing whether they are adequately cultivating their capabilities, and in turn, whether justice is being realised (Nussbaum 2006: 73).

Jennifer Ruger's work on global health inequalities has also embraced this emphasis on supporting individuals' 'beings and doings' through a concept of health capabilities (Ruger 2006). Global health inequalities are morally troubling here, because deprivations in the capability to function threaten individuals' well-being, defined as having capabilities to achieve a range of beings and doings, or the freedom to be what the individual wants to be and what he or she wants to do (Ruger 2006: 999). Justice requires that a society provides people 'with the necessary conditions for achieving the highest possible threshold level of health so they can have flourishing lives' (Ruger 2006: 1002). In a related vein, in proposing a moral framework to guide future progress toward the Millennium Development Goals, for example, Jeffrey Waage and his colleagues argue for a view of development as 'a dynamic process involving sustainable and equitable access to improved well-being . . . that is, the freedom to enjoy various combinations of beings and doings . . . [or] to make choices and act effectively' (Waage, Banjeri and Campbell 2010: 1009).

I want to suggest that the aims of enabling theories of justice, while ostensibly among the most well-suited for responding to global health inequities, suffer from an impoverished conception of the targets of the work of justice. They do so because they fail to reckon *fully* with our locatedness (both structural and spatial), interdependence and temporality. I argue that an ecological understanding of subjects offers a less idealised and more lived conception that can better inform ethical norms to guide work toward global health equity and, by better theorising their relationship to responsibility-bearers, motivate and assign responsibilities.

ECOLOGICAL SUBJECTS AND ETHICAL PLACE-MAKING

Enlivening and enriching the conception of the person found in much liberal moral and political philosophy that emphasises rationality, independence or self-reliance, and that assumes equality among us, Nussbaum, Young and Ruger each offer accounts of subjects that acknowledge our embodiment, our social nature, and the presence of social, economic, health and other inequities that generate ethically unacceptable vulnerabilities among us. Nussbaum's capabilities approach is perhaps the most explicit on these elements of subjectivity and their significance for justice. Nussbaum seeks acknowledgement of the 'many types of dignity in the world' (Nussbaum 2006: 54) by calling for a more Aristotelian, less Kantian image of the person, and 'bringing the rational and the animal into a more intimate relation with one another' (Nussbaum 2006: 54), and citing as her eighth principle of justice that care for children, the ill and the elderly 'should be a prominent focus of the world community', given its essential role in nurturing the capabilities (Nussbaum 2006: 321).

Yet for each of these theorists, the emphasis on the self in articulating the ideals of global justice serves to obscure our interdependence and need for caring relations (Tronto 1993; Kittay 2002). In a global economic order marked by the retraction of the public sector and a growing emphasis on individual responsibility for self-care and care of loved ones, upholding self-development and self-determination as ideals should give us pause. Additionally, their emphasis on individual choice and activity, including 'striving', 'achievement' and 'transformation', may eclipse other possibilities for the substance of a good life. I say more on this below. And even though references to activities such as 'development' and 'striving' suggest some acknowledgement of our temporal nature, the emphasis on 'being' (that is, well-being) might serve to obscure the fact that we, our relations and interactions, and the social, economic and political processes in which we are embedded, have a past and are ongoing, opening into the future under ever-changing conditions. We need a conception of the person that reckons more fully and explicitly with the significance of the body, our social, interdependent nature and temporality, and that points to 'a fundamental role of all societies [viz.] to provide the circumstances under which humans can be cared for and thrive, given their differing degrees of frailty and vulnerability' over time and through change (Kittay 2002: 78).

Still, this is not the whole story for embodied, interdependent subjects. 'Place matters for health', assert researchers in societal determinants (Laveist, Gaskin and Trujillo 2011). *Places* have to meet certain conditions, indeed, if subjects are to survive, not to mention realise justice. Rosemarie Garland-Thomson's notion of the 'misfit' helps to shed light on the idea. Our shared vulnerability is not, she argues, just in our embodiment and potential to suffer, but in the need for 'fit' between our bodies and our environments. 'Misfits' are those who are ensconced in environments that cannot sustain them, or when, as she puts it, 'the world fails the flesh' (Garland-Thomson 2010). To address injustice, then, we need an account that reckons more thoroughly with the relationship between the embodiment and implacement – structural and spatial – of interdependent, asymmetrically vulnerable subjects.[1] Subjects cannot survive or thrive, for example, in the absence of functioning, effective public-health and healthcare systems and care relations, and they may struggle to do so when environments – social, institutional and other – are impoverished, constituted to narrowly define their possibilities and/or constrain their abilities to meet their needs and the needs of their loved ones. Thinking this way suggests that we should be wary of an excessive emphasis on individuals as the primary focus of efforts aimed at justice and health equity. Such efforts cannot be lucidly conceived apart from people's interdependence and their embeddedness in movement through social (often transnational) processes and places. I expand on this point below.

Now if we go further and consider the relationship between our interdependence and 'implacement', we find ourselves reflecting on what geographers have called the 'intersubjectivity' of identities and place. Seeing *place* in relational terms – that is, as *intersubjectively constructed* – 'highlights the multiplicity of locations as well as the variety of interactions between people who are located differently that go into making places' (Raghuram, Madge and Noxolo 2009: 8). This is significant ethically because it raises questions about *responsibilities* 'for those relations with other parts of the world through which . . . identit[ies] are formed' (Massey 2004: 13). As Massey argues, to the extent that we are 'constitutively, elements within a wider, configurational, distributed geography . . . that raises a second question [concerning] the geography of relations through which any particular identity is established and maintained' (Massey 2006: 93).

Consider two examples of the intersubjectivity of identity and place that centre on the migration of care-workers and the consequent deepening of global health inequities. Joan Tronto has argued that the tendency among middle-class and more affluent families in the United States to understand caring in private terms – that is, as a matter involving the needs of their loved ones exclusively and including such activities as hiring nannies or home care-workers – can lead to moral hazards, including social harm. 'In a competitive society,' she observes, 'what it means to care well for one's own [family] is to make sure that they have a competitive edge against other [families]' (Tronto 2006: 10). More privileged people may not be concerned if the caring needs of those who provide them with services go unmet. Ultimately, those acting with what Tronto describes as 'privileged irresponsibility' 'ignore the ways in which their own caring activities [often against a background of weak social support for family care needs] continue to perpetuate inequality' (Tronto 2006: 13). This invites reflection on how identities are connected through the transnational division of care labour, and how health stands to be adversely affected and inequities perpetuated in places confronting care deficits and absent or eroding care infrastructure.

Turning to the second example, post-colonial theorists maintain that conversations on the topic of care-worker migration tend to obscure the extent to which this 'draws upon colonial legacies to make up the postcolonial present', which serves to 'disavow ... the interdependent relationships ... established over centuries of co-production of medical care across different parts of the Empire' (Raghuram 2009: 30), relationships that can generate injustice over time to the extent that they expand possibilities for some while contracting them for others. With major capital at stake, indebted governments in low-income countries have been in recent decades 'only too eager to provide this *habitat* [my emphasis]' for producing health care-workers, especially nurses, determined by cost-benefit analyses to be valuable as export to labour markets in more affluent nations, even when their own health-care needs go unmet (Tolentino 1996: 53; Lorenzo, Galvez-Tan and Icamina 2007). Here again, identities and places are intersubjectively constructed and maintained, with implications for health equity.

This notion of the intersubjectivity of identities and place enriches conceptions of justice put forward by moral philosophers like Thomas Pogge and Iris Marion Young that emphasise our relationships to the injustices others suffer – including health inequities – in grounding global responsibilities. These approaches all identify dense structural social and economic relationships between people around the world – relationships that systematically privilege some at the same time they oppress others – as bases for obligations of justice. For Thomas Pogge, by 'shaping and enforcing the social conditions that foreseeably and avoidably cause the monumental suffering of global poverty, we are harming the global poor' (Pogge 2004: 33). On this view, our connection is a matter of being 'materially involved' in or 'substantially contributing to' upholding the institutions responsible for injustice (Pogge 2004: 137). Young proposes a 'social connection model of responsibility' in which 'obligations of justice arise between [agents] by virtue of the social processes that connect them' (Young 2006: 102).

Relational conceptions of justice highlight a range of contributors to global health inequities. I mention only a few to highlight the thick interconnections between countries when it comes to the global health workforce. Underdevelopment in the global South and the emergence of neo-liberal economic policies may be the greatest contributor. International financial institutions, chiefly the World Bank and International Monetary Fund (IMF), under the influence of dominant countries such as the United States, have compelled low-income

countries to balance budgets and become more competitive players
in the global marketplace using structural adjustment policies, which
have in many places led to reductions in employment, including health
sector employment (Buchan, Parkin and Sochalski 2003; Stillwell et al.
2004). Many people in lower-income countries are thus driven to seek
work in richer nations with governments being dependent upon the
remittances they send back home (http://web.worldbank.org/WBSITE/
EXTERNAL/TOPICS/0..contentMDK:21924020~pagePK:5105988
~piPK:360975~theSitePK:214971,00.html). Some, like the Philippines,
actively recruit and train their own citizens for export to labour markets
in high-income countries, including health care-workers who go
abroad as part of the country's economic development plans (Lorenzo
et al. 2007; Rodriguez 2008). At the same time, healthcare industry
organisations in high-income countries, who regard international
recruitment as a way to address health workforce shortages and at the
same time keep hiring costs down and improve retention, often lobby
for an easing of immigration requirements in order to gain access to
skilled health care-workers from abroad (Connell and Stillwell 2006).

These and other policies and practices carried out by governments,
international lending bodies, the for-profit sector and others, reflect our
complex, dense interdependence, that is, our intersubjectivity when it
comes to identity and place; they also create, sustain and deepen global
health inequities by eroding capacities for care in low-income countries, rendering them places of deprivation. As Iris Young puts it: even
when geographically distant, we *'dwell* [my emphasis] together . . .
within a set of problems and relationships of structural interdependence' (Young 2000: 197).

This set of arguments concerning intersubjectivity and responsibility
finds articulation in Lorraine Code's work. Code 'proposes a way of
engaging . . . with the implications of patterns, places, and the interconnections of lives and events in and across the human and nonhuman
world' (Code 2006: 4). An ecological analysis situates knowledge-
production efforts in particular places, and further, conceives of these
as 'intersecting' 'with other locations and their occupants' (Code 2006:
21). The ecological subject herein is an embodied creature for whom
'locatedness [socially *and* spatially] and interdependence are integral to
its possibilities'. Ecological subjects, as Code puts it, are 'made by and
mak[e our] relations in reciprocity with other subjects *and* [my empha-
sis] with . . . (multiple, diverse) locations' (Code 2006: 128). The inspir-

ing aim of ecological thinking is to 'discern conditions for mutually sustaining lives within a specific locality . . . or *the interrelations among them* [my emphasis]' (Code 2006: 60–1) and 'to enact principles of ideal cohabitation' (Code 2006: 24).

In light of these reflections, I suggest first that we should jettison the excessive emphasis in enabling conceptions of justice on self, being and notions of achievement and mastery. If, instead, we focus our attention on the idea that we are profoundly social, interdependent, variably vulnerable subjects with a temporal, generative nature, we could perhaps describe justice as enablement through the concepts of 'becoming' and 'enduring' (Bergson 1911); that is, on this view, our capacities for becoming and enduring in cohabitation. Becoming can be understood as having the capacity for processes of development, evolution and expansion (Grosz 1999). Enduring or duration encompasses capacities for sustaining ongoing processes of 'conservation, resilience, preservation, and abiding' (Casey 1999: 218).[2] Decision, action and mastery are not necessarily – though they could very well be – what gives life meaning and value for subjects. The concepts of becoming and duration leave open more possibilities. Both unfold over time. Each of them can occur only in concert with other subjects. Moreover, each can be precarious, or perhaps impossible, depending on how subjects are situated in social, political and economic structures, and in particular geographic locations or 'habitats'.

Further, I want to suggest that responsibility for justice in global health might best be conceived as involving 'ethical place-making' (Raghuram, Madge and Noxolo 2009: 7; Massey 2006) for ecological subjects, dwelling in relations of mutual sustenance. Thoroughly fleshing out the meaning of this notion of 'ethical place-making' – coined by geographers – and its significance for global health equity warrants a separate project. Here I offer a mere sketch.

Place, at least on philosophical accounts, 'is no fixed thing' (Casey 1997: 286). It can be understood as being *around* us, as the commonsense (and public health) view has it, but also *in* and *with* us. That is to say, *place* may refer to geographic regions, neighbourhoods and communities, and built places such as institutional care settings and workplaces – the focus of much research on societal determinants of health – but also bodies and psyches. Jacques Derrida, with an architectural notion of place as involving the movement of time-bounded bodies, speaks of 'scenographies of passage' where 'passage connotes movement between places [and] . . . a place *through which* to pass' (Casey 1997: 313). We might also draw insight from the notion, developed by Gilles Deleuze and Felix Guattari, of 'nomad space' to capture the experience of those, such as migrants, who are in some sense distributed between places, who are at once 'here/there *and* there/here' (Casey 1997: 305), and who often see themselves as having 'a foot here, a foot there, a foot *nowhere* [my emphasis]' (DiCicco-Bloom 2004: 28). Thinking ecologically also reveals the need to take seriously the 'rhizomatic[3] structure of [our] implacement' (Casey 1997: 337); that is, the reality that our locatedness involves the continual navigation of a set of relations between places: homes, places of work, care settings, borders and so on. Ecological subjects can suffer ill-health as a result of social structures and processes that create fragmentation or cause rupture, as in lived experiences of segregation, movement between care settings, hypermobility, migration and familial separation.

An account of justice for global health that reckons with our implacement calls, then, for situating ecological subjects within and between particular yet interconnected places around the world where the ill and dependent and those who care for them dwell – homes, places of work, institutional care settings, recruiting offices, immigration facilities and so on – and making more equal the conditions therein that support becoming and duration. This means, more specifically, refraining from creating conditions of deprivation (that is, conditions that cannot support and sustain capacities for becoming and enduring); supporting conditions that facilitate and sustain becoming and duration; and promoting conditions for ending deprivation and facilitating and sustaining becoming and duration. Justice, it must be underscored, cannot be realised merely by refraining from interference or avoiding the imposition of systems or orders that prevent others from achieving opportunities. It requires active intervention.

To take an example, consider the asymmetrical, that is, low-income to high-income country, migration of health care-workers. Destination countries on this view have responsibilities to design policies that avoid the active recruitment of care-workers from low-income countries with high disease burdens and health-worker shortages; to support efforts to train, employ and retain the health workforce in countries from which workers migrate, as well as efforts to ensure access to health-care for populations in source countries suffering under shortages;

to support the development of alternative imaginaries and channels of opportunity for girls coming-of-age in current care-worker export zones; to promote greater investment in the healthcare workforce of destination countries, especially in health sectors with major shortages, such as long-term care and rural care, to avoid persistent problems with recruitment and retention. If we embrace such an alternative moral ontology and think of ourselves – as individuals and states – less as independent and self-contained or loosely connected, or, worse, polarised, and instead start from notions of embodied subjects situated in interdependent habitats and networks of responsibility and care (Robinson 2006; Sevenhuijsen et al. 2006), the potential for global justice, including global justice in health, seems far more ripe.

THE BENEFITS OF AN ETHIC OF PLACE-MAKING

The ecological subject is only 'a distant relative' of the disembodied, unlocated and unlocatable, 'interchangeable' subject that appears in liberal moral and political theory (Code 2006: 5) and that haunts many policy discussions. By reckoning with our embodied and socio-spatially situated nature, this account resists tendencies to privilege particular, culturally dominant, conceptions of persons and their most vital capacities and instead allows for paying careful attention to particularities of people and places. It allows for contextually sensitive explorations of how it is and should be for ecological subjects in the many places they inhabit and traverse, striving to become and endure. Because for ecological subjects, meanings and expressions of becoming and enduring, of harm and so forth, are situated socially and constituted relationally (Miller 2009), robust, egalitarian decision-making processes and responsive institutions and interactions are necessary to determine what precisely is needed in particular places for particular people; that is, justice demands fair processes for asking what would ethical place-making mean here, or here, or here?

With the capacities to 'become' and 'endure' as universal norms and egalitarian processes for deciding on their precise content, indeed, we can avoid a kind of neo-colonialism offered with a caring face. When it comes to the ill and dependent, self-determination and self-transformation may be especially dangerous ideals in an environment of cost-cutting, in that it may well leave them vulnerable to some notion that they can be left to fend for themselves when it comes to their care needs. In a culture already marked by an emphasis on self-reliance, this seems perfectly likely. When countries are described as 'developing', the implication is that they are behind and working to 'catch up'. This framing suggests that people globally are in some sort of queue, obscuring the relations of inequality that generate and perpetuate deprivation and suppress ideas about alternative futures (Massey 2006). Under the banner of self-development and self-determination, global economic structures have already imperilled, and stand to further imperil, the ill and dependent, and many of those who care for them, through the 'shifting of responsibility for social risks onto [them as] individuals, and transforming [what had been understood as social] responsibility into a problem of self-care' (Schild 2007: 199).

Moreover, to the extent that received accounts of global justice, including arguments focused on global health equity, use *well-being* and *flourishing* interchangeably, the proposal here calling instead for us to embrace the concepts of becoming and duration seems appropriately ambitious in not aiming at the higher ideal of flourishing but taking seriously prospects greater than mere subsistence. Identifying norms that can be discussed and institutionalised sooner rather than later seems crucial, given the severity of the injustice some people face under contemporary conditions (Parekh 2008: 107).

Maybe most important, the recognition in this account of the inter-subjectivity of place offers new resources for grounding responsibilities for global justice. While most accounts point to our shared humanity, feelings of compassion or benevolence for others (Nussbaum 2006; Gould 2007a, 2007b), or our participation in processes that generate injustice (Pogge 2004; Young 2006), ecological thinking offers a more robust way of understanding our connections under globalisation. We should accept responsibilities for justice and for global health equity not merely because of our shared humanity, our feelings for others or our contribution to injustice, but also because of who and what we are as ecological subjects: creatures whose identities and dwelling places are not merely relational, but intersubjectively constructed, indeed, mutually constitutive.

What we find, then, by thinking ecologically, is that even where the governments and citizenry of wealthy countries, along with other agents whose policies and practices have global reach, are not motivated as this and other authors are by moral arguments, especially those that ground responsibilities in our connections to injustice, they may be moved by *prudential* arguments that acknowledge our inter-dependence. Consider again the case of health care-worker migra-tion: such agents have prudential reasons to be concerned about the health status of care-workers, their education and training, and their treatment under labour and immigration policies. And because not all health care-workers trained abroad emigrate, the local populations in source countries *may* benefit if the healthcare infrastructure in these countries meets high standards for education and training. Although this is not the richest or even an accurate interpretation of intersubjec-tivity, given urgent realities on the ground, especially in low-income countries, this minimalist view may at least begin to encourage greater appreciation for our profound interdependence.[4] Ecological thinking, at minimum then, strengthens the case for prudentially motivated action aimed at global health equity. In its more robust interpretation, it enriches relational conceptions of justice by showing how profound our connections truly are.

Yet another benefit of thinking ecologically is that, by being able to trace more precisely the connections between those who contribute to and suffer from injustice, we are in a better position to assign responsi-bilities whose nature and extent vary. 'Differences in kind and degree' of responsibilities 'correlate with an agent's position within the struc-tural processes' (Young 2006: 126). The questions for justice concern how we are connected and what are our capacities.

Finally, an approach to global health equity that focuses on the mutual sustenance of places that support capacities for becoming and enduring strikes the right balance between acknowledging the past and privileging the future. In its very structure, it aims at ensuring a future, indeed, a more equitable one. This would represent a major advance in global public health policy and planning. As critics have observed, the future is strikingly absent from view (Graham 2010). At the same time, on this view we see more clearly the relationship between the past, present and future, and so can hold those who have contributed to injustice accountable for past wrongs so they can contribute to justice in the future. The moral attitude is not so much one of blame, which could undermine efforts to address injustice through its more adversarial posture (Young 2006), but rather acknowledgement and (inevitably situated) engaged reflection on our ongoing connections. It invites us to ask not just 'what has been done?' but also 'what has not been done?' (Young 2004a: 376).

Notes

1. Edward Soja (1989) describes a 'spatialized ontology'.
2. I grant that there may be pejorative connotations with the concept *enduring*. Here I hope to avoid the association of surviving unrelenting hardship.
3. According to the *Oxford American Dictionary* (1980), a rhizome is 'a root-like stem growing along or under the ground sending out both roots and shoots' (779).
4. I am indebted to Ryoa Chung and Christine Straehle for helping me develop this line of argument.

Chapter 4

HEALTH INEQUALITIES, CAPABILITIES AND GLOBAL JUSTICE

Sridhar Venkatapuram

The interest in the ethics of health *inequalities* rather than just health or healthcare is becoming more widespread and gaining momentum. In particular, health researchers and others concerned about the social determinants and social gradients (that is, inequalities) of preventable ill-health and premature mortality are increasingly drawing on the normative domain of social ethics and justice. At the same time, political philosophers are extending their traditional scope of concern about social justice and inequality into the domain of health. Ethical evaluation of *global* health inequalities, then, requires integrating reasoning across empirical health sciences and normative ethics and extending the scope to include all societies and the entire human species. While this description may initially suggest a two-step – first domestic, then global – reasoning process, it is not only plausible but perhaps logically and ethically necessary that both empirical and normative analyses of health and health inequalities require starting with a global perspective.

The flip side of the ethics of (global) health inequalities being of interest to diverse actors and encompassing diverse concerns is that discussions can cut across each other, misunderstandings across disciplines or the research versus policy divide can give rise to antipathies, not to mention that a wide range of philosophical and ethical issues as well as related ambiguities become enmeshed. The joining up of health, inequality and ethics increases complexity multiplicatively rather than additively. For example, while stark numerical inequalities in health outcomes may initially provoke moral indignation, why exactly are health inequalities a moral worry? Is it because of the inequality in suffering, or because the numbers evidence the preventable suffering of some? Are health inequalities instantiations of inequalities of some more abstract goods such as 'life chances'? Or are health inequalities a worry because they are uniquely morally troublesome? That is, is health unique or a 'special moral good' whose inequality raises distinct ethical concerns? Indeed, even if health is special, is it the fact of inequality *per se* that is the worry, or because health has some other instrumental use? Moreover, is any type of inequality bad or are some inequalities worse or better than others?

Such questions seeking to identify whether health, some other good or inequality is the more dominant, guiding concern may seem like navel-gazing to non-philosophers and especially exasperating to those who are anxious to alleviate visible suffering, impairments or prevent deaths of human beings. Indeed, there is a commonly recognised moral duty to uphold the 'rule of rescue', or to act when there is a feasible possibility to avert serious harm or death (McKie and Richardson 1982). However, when preventable impairments and premature mortality are an enduring reality and not just a one-off event, after a few steps into taking action various difficult decisions will bring us back to these original questions.

Consider the example of the Bill & Melinda Gates Foundation. It is an unprecedented global actor in the sphere of public health: just its annual giving toward health programmes is almost equal to the entire annual operating budget of the World Health Organization. Yet, the foundation is both commended for its support of programmes addressing HIV/AIDS or maternal mortality in developing countries as well as criticised for its motives, for who runs the foundation, what work it does, how it does the work, which organisations it supports, where it does it, and so forth. Such divergent responses to the foundation's functioning show that alongside a 'rule of rescue' principle that motivates those running the Gates foundation and many of us to act quickly in the face of preventable human suffering, there is also a pressing need to step back and think much harder about the philosophy and ethics of enduring ill-health and health inequalities, within and across countries. There are plenty of other real-world examples of vigorous disagreements about the who, what, where, when, why and how of social responses to health issues, domestically and globally, which are fundamentally rooted in whether health, some other good and/or inequality in some form is the driving concern – when they are a concern at all.

Helpfully, when it comes to thinking harder about global health inequalities, a number of political philosophers have already provided much insight. The moral concern for the 'global poor' underlying current global justice debates most often starts with the concern over the scale of their premature deaths and high levels of impairments. Low life expectancies of populations and inequalities in life expectancies across countries are often the first facts presented, and said to raise moral dilemmas to do with (global) justice. However, these facts are not presented as raising moral problems regarding health and justice. Instead, the focus is largely on premature mortality or life expectancy. Often implicitly, while sidestepping the issue of health, life expectancy is treated as the 'absolutist core' of human well-being. And like the equal moral worth of every human being, premature mortality as a moral bad is treated as something not needing explanation or justification; it is something that is assumed to resonate with the moral intuitions of most individuals who may hold a wide variety of philosophical views about justice. From there, reasoning is presented for the ethical claims all human beings can make about their well-being, or for the scope of obligations to the well-being of foreigners (Brock 2005; Nussbaum 2006; Singer 2004). Some have identified the causal role of non-domestic actors in premature deaths and impairments of the 'global poor' and the relevant moral obligations (Pogge 2002). And, indeed, some philosophers have also made arguments that while stark health inequalities across societies may be a moral worry, they do not necessarily have to do with justice (Nagel 2005; Daniels 2008).

The focus on absolute levels and relative inequalities of life expectancies, and therefore, unavoidably health, being the starting point and driving motivation of global justice theorising fits well with the central aim of this chapter, which is to present a capabilities approach to reasoning about health inequalities and global justice. The capabilities approach, within discussions about social justice, is an approach that focuses on protecting and promoting the abilities of individuals to be and do valuable things in their lives – their freedoms. And, I would argue that life expectancy and health being the starting point of global justice debates is significantly due to the influence the capabilities approach and its advocates have had on contemporary debates on justice, particularly through their arguments for making the idea of justice relevant to the daily lives of the worst-off individuals in the world.

The chapter proceeds as follows. Section 1 provides some relevant background by discussing the three-tier 'health equity' principles well known in public health literature as well as the parallel 'equality of what' debates in political philosophy. Section 2 discusses some different approaches to valuing health, and the far reach of the concern for health and health equity in light of social determinants of health research. Section 3 describes the argument for the moral entitlement to the capability to be healthy and implications for global justice. Section 4 concludes. My modest aim in this chapter is to provide an overview of how the capabilities approach relates to discussions on health equity, equality and justice, and global justice. I do not attempt to provide a comprehensive argument or defence (see chapters by Yukiko Asada and Phillip Cole for alternative accounts of the capabilities approach to global health concerns).

1. HEALTH EQUITY AND 'EQUALITY OF WHAT' DEBATES

Starting in the late 1980s, the term 'health equity' began to appear more frequently in health research literature and policy discussions. It presently functions as an umbrella term that captures both the concern about the persistence of preventable ill-health and health inequalities across social groups in industrialised countries, as well as the concern about the persistent high prevalence of preventable mortality and impairments in poor countries (Evans et al. 2001; Whitehead 1990; Braveman 2006; Braveman and Gruskin 2003). This is remarkable because historically health issues facing rich versus poor countries have been seen as requiring fundamentally different analytical paradigms and responses, a notion shaped by theories of demographic and epidemiological transitions (Omran 1971; Preston 2007). While some may attribute the current joining up of the health concerns facing both industrialised and developing countries to the process of globalisation or the emergence of 'global health', there is also a more prosaic explanation.

Margaret Whitehead initially developed a conception of health equity for the World Health Organization's Europe office in the late 1980s. The motivating idea behind Whitehead's conception of health equity is that certain ethical values compel social action to decrease 'health inequities' across social groups. Because all health impairments, including the ultimate impairment of death, are not necessarily morally troubling, to identify the subset of all health *inequalities* which qualify as *inequities* that require a social response as a matter of social justice, three criteria are identified in the form of a decision tree (Whitehead

1990). A health difference or inequality becomes a health inequity when it is deemed to be (a) avoidable, (b) unnecessary and (c) unfair or unjust. A society is morally obligated to act to prevent and mitigate the health inequities that remain after applying the three-tier filter (Evans et al. 2001; Whitehead 1990, 1992). The success in applying the health equity concept to the broad diversity of countries and regions within the European community in the 1990s made it plausible to generalise it to all the countries in the world.

Whitehead's effort to bridge health sciences and normative social ethics was pioneering and the principles have gained wide international acceptance. However, the criteria have a number of conceptual weaknesses. The most prominent weakness is the overarching ambiguity about whether the moral concern about health inequalities is only regarding the distribution patterns of health constraints – inequalities between social groups – or also includes other dimensions. Should we be morally troubled primarily about relative health *inequalities* between groups, or that some groups have poor health, or that some groups are not achieving what they could – which is evidenced through a comparison with what other groups are achieving? And importantly, are we worried about inter-group inequalities, inter-individual inequalities, or both?

These ambiguities about whether our ethical evaluation of health inequalities should be driven foremost by the concern for *equality* or the value of health (*priority*), or both, and whether the ethical concern is for groups or individuals, or both, are not minor issues. It is crucially important to be clear about them from the beginning as the particular choices made profoundly determine much of the reasoning that follows (Parfit 1997; Murray et al. 1999; Gakidou et al. 2000; Braveman et al. 2000, 2001; Asada 2007).

I have discussed the many ambiguities about the three health equity principles in more detail elsewhere (Venkatapuram 2011a; Venkatapuram and Marmot 2009). What is worth restating here is that fairness and justice cannot be the last of the considerations. When the criterion of 'fairness and justice' is considered third and last, after avoidability and necessity, the people with health constraints that become classified as 'unavoidable' or 'necessary' by the first two steps are pushed outside the scope of justice. That is, no claims from justice are available to individuals who experience 'unavoidable' or 'necessary' impairments and mortality. This is hugely problematic. The social response to individuals who are vulnerable to or experience unavoidable impairments (that is, genetic diseases) or necessary impairments or mortality (necessary for what?) cannot just be silence. Nor is it acceptable for their claims to be postponed for being 'hard cases' or handled as a matter for charity (Kittay 1997; Wasserman 2006; Nussbaum 2006). Nowhere else more than when we are dealing with social decisions about life and death of individuals does the respect for the equal moral worth of every person have to be recognised and accounted for in a meaningful way. Especially the notion that impairments and mortality of some individuals are 'necessary' requires extraordinary justification. It cannot be pre-supposed to be a simple criterion or accepted so easily as it is done within the traditional health equity literature.

Even if we were to accept justice and fairness as the last consideration, current advocates of the three-tier criteria express no clear commitment to a particular conception of justice or fairness. There are references to human rights, and oblique references to Rawlsian social justice, and even to the capabilities approach (Peter and Evans 2001; Anand 2002; Braveman and Gruskin 2003; Ostlin and Diderichsen 2001). And, despite the use of human rights rhetoric by health equity advocates, which directly admits them into discussions about global justice, the three-pronged view is actually unsympathetic to rights. Health equity advocates would probably have great difficulty navigating the conflicts between rights, and unlikely to side with the individual in the classic conflict between individual rights and increasing overall social benefit. That is, decreasing the magnitude of health inequities is likely to be given priority over respecting a particular individual's right to health or other human rights. In fact, some human rights are clearly violated by the first two criteria, and what rights or claims individuals are left with after the last criterion is unclear. Nevertheless, despite the various weaknesses and ambiguities in the health equity principles, their catalysing role in engendering much greater attention to the normative dimensions of health inequalities should be praiseworthy.

Equality of What?

In contrast to the health equity criteria's exclusive focus on health inequalities and ambiguity regarding individual claims, parallel discussions in political philosophy have been considering the ethics of inequalities in a broad range of moral goods or 'spaces', and specifically in relation to the claims of individuals. Indeed, the concern with equality and inequality has been a central theme in moral and political philosophy for most of the twentieth century and into the twenty-first. And, while there is no self-evident logical relation between equality and social justice (another central topic of political philosophy), a common starting point is that for any conception or theory of liberal social justice to be plausible in the modern world it has to treat human beings equally in some meaningful way (Sen 1996; Kane 1996a; Kane 1996b). To put an even finer point on it, to be taken seriously, contemporary theories of justice must not just express platitudes regarding the moral equality of persons but must treat individuals equally in some substantive way that is relevant to the theory (Sen 1982a). Such a starting point, however, does not identify in what space or how societies should treat individuals equally. And, as evidenced in the current debates on global justice, there is much disagreement about whether such a starting point means that every extant human being must be treated equally in a meaningful way within the scope of a theory of social justice.

In a seminal 1979 paper titled 'Equality of What', Amartya Sen interrogates the place of equality in different theories or approaches to social justice including utilitarianism, and theories that distribute resources such as John Rawls' famous theory which distributes 'primary goods' (Sen 1982a). Sen argues that both types of approach should be rejected by showing how their focal points of equality directly offend our moral intuitions, their implications in certain situations run counter to our moral intuitions, or they run counter to some other more basic moral principles. Sen goes on to argue for 'basic capability equality'. That is, rather than the target of equality being related to mental states such as in utilitarianism or the amounts of different resources, Sen avers that our normative evaluations should focus on freedoms – on what individuals are able to be and do in their lives. In subsequent publications, Sen continues to develop the idea of equality of basic capabilities while also rejecting other approaches to social justice such as libertarian theories that focus on *equal rights* or those that locate equality in their equal guarantees for *basic income* or satisfying *basic needs* (Sen 1982b, Sen 1997b, Sen, 1981).

Despite Sen's formidable arguments over three decades rejecting the most prominent approaches to social justice, and his constructive arguments in support of the capabilities approach, the equality of what debates are more active than ever. Some individuals have become convinced by Sen's arguments and motivated to extend further the capabilities approach theory or apply it in the real world. Others have become galvanised to identify new targets or defend their chosen approach to social justice against Sen's criticisms. Some have even pursued the strategy of showing how their chosen approach with a few tweaks becomes very similar to the capabilities approach. Amid such prodigious philosophical activity it is, however, worth noting that John Rawls, the most pre-eminent modern philosopher of social justice, responds to Sen's arguments by stating that capabilities are essential to explain the propriety of his own focal points of equality, or 'primary goods'; that primary goods pre-suppose basic capability equality (Rawls 1999: 13).

In any case, myriad focal points of equality are presently being advanced including rights, welfare, advantage, resources, capabilities, opportunities for welfare and mid-fare. And each of these focal points is attached to a further myriad of distributive rules including absolute equality, priority, sufficiency, maximisation, optimisation and shortfall equity. Justice, focal points of equality and distribution rules go together. As Elizabeth Anderson states so nicely, theories of justice have a metric and a rule (Anderson 2010).

While this is only a thumbnail sketch of equality and justice debates, it may now be understandable that what are deemed to be unjust inequalities vary according to a chosen theory's focal point of equality (*what*), and/or are a deviation from the correlative distribution rules – *how* the valued things are distributed and *to whom* they are distributed. At the same time, out of the foundational reasoning that develops a target of equality and its associated distribution rule(s) come moral rights and claims. That is, the substantive moral claims or rights individuals have within each theory are supervenient on the theory's reasoning about the focal point of equality and the distribution rule(s). Individuals have rights to the focal points of equality and their distribution rules. To paraphrase Norman Daniels, rights or claims are the moral fruits that are harvested from theories of justice (Daniels 2008: 15). And this is why a simple list of rights, such as human rights, even when enshrined in law, without a background theory does not convince. And why a rights approach is unable to offer guidance in responding to the conflicts of rights and other wicked problems.

One thing should strike as peculiar about modern philosophical discussions on equality and justice. In contrast to a broad array of focal points of equality such as income, utility or civil liberties, because of their link to human well-being the debates have only very recently begun to consider health as a target. Some may ask, like Sen does, how can health not but be central to social justice and equity (Sen 2002)? At least two reasons may explain the long absence of health. First, many prominent participants of the equality of what debates have held certain assumptions about health, its causes and distribution. For example, John Rawls understands human health to be a 'natural good' and subject to random luck over the life course; he sees health as not something significantly or directly socially produced, so it does not even come within the scope of social justice, let alone that it is central to it (Rawls 1971: 62; Rawls 1993: 20).

The second reason has to do with the conceptual architecture prevalent in political philosophy. For example, in social contract theories, theorising about justice requires certain pre-requisite 'circumstances of justice'. Rawls, following David Hume, identifies these as (a) moderate scarcity of resources in order for social co-operation to be seen as possible and necessary; (b) rough equality of persons so that no one can dominate another; and (c) self-interested individuals (since impartially benevolent individuals would make justice superfluous). Moreover, the agents of justice also require some idealising assumptions. Once again, in Rawls' case, agents are imagined to have the capacity to reason, possess a sense of justice, and importantly, they are healthy over the entire life span. Such structures of ideal theorising erase both certain kinds of people as well as pressing issues in the lives of most human beings. Children and those severely impaired are erased because they are seen as not having full capacity to reason. And, by assuming healthy individuals, all concerns relating to the causes, levels, relative distribution, consequences, persistence through generations, burden on care-givers and so forth are also erased.

In light of the absence of health in justice debates, Norman Daniels' theory of justice and healthcare was indeed pioneering (Daniels 1985). While keeping Rawls' theory of justice architecture intact, Daniels extends it to include an explicit concern for health. He argues that health is an important determinant of equality of opportunity, one of Rawls' focal points of equality. Daniels then proceeds to argue that, therefore, healthcare broadly conceived should be a basic entitlement. Moreover, healthcare is to be distributed in such a way that ensures individuals *maintain* 'species typical functioning' (health) in order to ensure they have fair equality of opportunity, given talents and skills, to pursue the normal range of life plans prevalent in a given society. Daniels recently amended his theory partly in light of learning of the robust relationship between wider social arrangements and health outcomes in addition to access to healthcare (Daniels 2008). I discuss social determinants of health below but first focus on how different theories of social justice value health.

2. VALUING HEALTH DIFFERENTLY, AND THE FAR REACH OF THE CONCERN FOR HEALTH

What is noteworthy in Daniels' argument is that health has value primarily because it is an important determinant of equality of opportunity. Health inequalities are a worry because of their role in producing inequalities in opportunity to pursue a normal range of life plans. In contrast, for utilitarians, being in good health relates to states of being or functioning that produce positive mental states or utility. Here too, health is valued for its instrumental role. Health inequalities are a worry only *insofar as* they are decreasing the maximal amount of welfare in a population. As long as maximal utility is achieved, inequalities in health are not a worry.

In comparison to these previous two accounts, in the capabilities approach, health is both intrinsically and instrumentally valuable. Being in good health partly constitutes well-being, a valued state of being. So it is intrinsically valuable. Being in good health also makes possible the planning, pursuing and revising of life plans. So it is also instrumentally valuable. Inequalities in health are ethically troublesome because of the distinct nature of health as a basic component of well-being, and because of its profound determining role in other valuable capabilities. Perceptive readers may notice that Daniels' valuation of health for its role in equality of opportunity looks similar to the valuation of health capability. Capability is opportunity, so health capability is valuable for its role in creating opportunities. Yet, while Daniels' primary good of equality of opportunity to achieve a normal range of life plans and a capability could be similar ideas, a capability also has intrinsic value; a life of opportunity is a moral good in itself. Moreover, as I mentioned above, Rawls himself states that primary goods pre-suppose a whole variety of circumstances of justice, including basic capabilities. There are many further differences between Daniels' account of health and equality of opportunity versus a health capability (Venkatapuram 2011a). I will discuss the detailed construction of the capability to be healthy and the related moral claims in the next section. I focus now on making the point that once health is given value, in diverse ways by different theories of justice, the reach of social action may be surprisingly wide in order to realise such ethical value of health.

Health and Basic Social Arrangements

Over the last three decades, epidemiologists have produced compelling evidence that health outcomes (for example, life expectancy, mortality rates, obesity and cognitive development) are distributed along a social gradient; each socio-economic class – defined by income, occupational grade or educational attainment – has worse health outcomes than the one above it (Kawachi et al. 2002; Macintyre and Marmot 1997; Marmot et al. 1997). There is a health/illness gradient from top to bottom of the social hierarchy within societies. Research also shows that the steeper the socio-economic gradient (that is, more social inequality), the lower overall health and well-being of the entire population; everyone in that society is worse off in the domain of health and many other domains than they could be otherwise (Wilkinson and Pickett 2009; Deaton 2003). Of course, we have known for a long time that chronic ill-health and impairments also negatively affect economic resources and social position. But the causal effects in this direction do not come close to explaining the social distribution of life expectancy and all types of impairments.

The remarkable findings on the social gradient of ill-health have motivated numerous research studies on the underlying causal determinants. The important thing to note here is that, unlike studies which try to identify what causes a disease in one individual rather than another, these studies aim to identify what causes disease in certain individuals and in differing amounts in different social groups. The main hypothesis is that the causal factors are in the social conditions; the factors affecting social groups differently in different places on the social hierarchy. Where one stands on the social gradient determines the types and levels of harmful exposures and protective factors that lead to ill-health and mortality (additionally, as Ryoa Chung and Matthew R. Hunt argue in their chapter, disaster relief provision can serve to reinforce this social hierarchy).

The research has so far illuminated a whole range of social

determinants of ill-health over the entire life cycle, starting from the social conditions surrounding the mother while in-utero to quality of social relationships in old age. While availability of healthcare is crucial, other more influential causal determinants include such things as early infant care and stimulation, safe and secure employment, housing conditions, discrimination, self-respect, personal relationships, community cohesion and income inequality (Berkman and Kawachi 2000; Marmot and Wilkinson 1999). What is relevant to the reasoning about the scope of justice is that these determinants operate at levels ranging from the micro such as material deprivations and individual level psycho-social mechanisms to the macro such as community cultures, national political regimes, and global processes affecting trade and human rights.

Such social epidemiological research challenges both the prevailing individual level explanatory paradigm in epidemiology as well as social inaction or complacency regarding harmful social or 'structural' conditions domestically as well as globally. While the level of expenditures and quality of healthcare, individual behaviours and genetic risk factors clearly have a causal role, it is the social conditions that are most correlated with prevalence of preventable ill-health and mortality in a society. Such findings overwhelmingly motivate the understanding that mitigating preventable ill-health and premature mortality in individuals as well as their unequal social distribution (that is, inequalities) requires substantial changes to basic social institutions, processes, policies and values (Marmot 2006; Krieger and Birn 1998; Commission on Social Determinants of Health 2008).

The empirical research in social epidemiology thus extends the moral scope of the concern for health and health inequalities wide and deep into the basic structures of domestic and, indeed, global society. And many extant approaches to social justice are simply ill-equipped to evaluate the ethics of such a broad relationship between social and global arrangements and health/health inequalities. The assumptions and theoretical structures erase much of the health injustices or push these concerns outside the scope of justice. This is not so with the capabilities approach.

3. THE CAPABILITY TO BE HEALTHY

According to the capabilities approach, the metric of justice is capabilities; every human being has moral entitlements to various basic capabilities. Among these is a capability to be healthy (Venkatapuram 2011b; Sen 2009; Nussbaum 2011; Ruger 2010). More specifically, every human being has a moral entitlement to the *social bases* of an equitable capability to be healthy. Justice can require societies to do only what societies can, in fact, do. And equitability is a complex and evolving idea in the capabilities approach as well as more broadly in social justice debates. Nevertheless, the concepts of a moral right to basic capabilities, health as a basic capability and equitable capabilities take the capabilities approach a long way in reasoning about what the moral problem is regarding ill-health and health inequalities within and across countries, as well as regarding the components of an appropriate social response domestically and globally.

To show the coherence of a 'capability to be healthy', it may be best to start with what causes the thing called health. Every human being experiences different types and durations of physical and mental impairments, or different periods of health and illness, and lives for varying lengths of time due to the combined interactions of her internal biological endowments and needs, behaviours, external physical environment and social conditions (Evans and Stoddart 1990; Lalonde 1974). There is nothing controversial about such a descriptive statement. Interestingly, these four categories of causal factors of health and longevity are the same for a capability of an individual. A capability within the capabilities approach describes the substantive freedom or practical possibility of being or doing something X. Such practical possibility, in fact, reflects the interaction of an individual's internal biological and mental endowments and needs interacting with the external physical and social environment, and the person's behaviours or agency.

While we can accept that the determinants of health and of capability fall into four categories, there is the issue of how to relate health with capability as they clearly are not the same thing. Health can be conceived as the absence of disease, thus, seeing health capability as the capability to avoid disease, impairments and premature mortality. Or, if one finds the absence of disease and related notions incoherent, as I do, then health and health capability can also be positively conceived. Following Lennart Nordenfelt, I argue that health should be seen as a cluster of basic capabilities (Nordenfelt et al. 2001; Venkatapuram 2011a). More specifically, to be healthy is to be capable of doing and being some basic things that constitute a life with equal human dignity in the modern world.

A person's health capability clearly changes over the life cycle, and due to changes in the four causal categories of factors. And, as I stated above, the ethical claims to capabilities are actually to the social bases of the capability; they are claims to only what can be achieved through social action. Nevertheless, what Sen has been arguing for a long time, and what is now more widely appreciated through social epidemiology, is that the scope of social action is enormous (Sen 1998). Social conditions can directly influence internal biological pathways affecting health and longevity through individual psycho-social pathways and they can also function as 'causes of causes'; the cause that sets up the three other proximate determinants of health and longevity (that is, biology, environment, behaviours) (Marmot and Wilkinson 1999). Social arrangements profoundly determine who is actually born and their genetic endowments, how they behave, as well as the surrounding physical and social conditions. Therefore, an ethical claim to the social bases of the health capability has very wide reach.

So where do the ethical claims for health capability come from? Sen's arguments show that when equality is a fundamental social value, the logically correct focus of equality and justice should be capabilities. Aside from the value of equality, the basic value of human freedoms common to all human societies also gives rise to the claims to capabilities. Capabilities are types of freedoms, and basic capabilities are fundamental freedoms. In contrast, Nussbaum grounds the claims in human dignity. For her, as with many other philosophers, entitlement is implicit in the notion of dignity (Nussbaum 2006: 37). A life with human dignity entails certain threshold levels of activity and opportunity in various domains of living as a needy and sociable animal with the capacity to reason. She identifies ten such domains in terms of capabilities, of which two are the capabilities to live a full life span and to be healthy (Nussbaum 2006; Nussbaum 2011). Jennifer Prah Ruger also grounds capability claims in human flourishing and argues that individuals have a claim to the healthcare bases of 'central health capabilities'. This claim to healthcare, broadly conceived, extends to the point where a person reaches their unique biological limits or the highest known population average of health function in the world (Ruger 2010).

My own argument is that every human being has moral entitlement or a human right to the social bases of a sufficient and equitable capability to be healthy because of its intrinsic value in constituting human dignity as well as its instrumental value for conceiving, pursuing and revising one's own life plans within contemporary global society (Venkatapuram 2011a). The claim to a health capability is thus grounded in both fundamental social values of liberty and equality. And it is a Sen–Nussbaum 'hybrid' argument. The argument is grounded in both the Senian value of freedoms and Nussbaum's normative for argument for pre-political entitlements to basic capabilities, or what I define as health meta-capability. That is, health is a meta- or overarching capability to achieve or exercise a cluster of basic and inter-related capabilities and functionings, such as Nussbaum's ten central human capabilities (Nussbaum 2011; Nordenfelt 2012; Venkatapuram 2012).

Capabilities Justice and Global Health Inequalities

The conceptual problem of global justice for many is formulated as the question of whether there are any ethical obligations owed to foreigners, and if so, what kind, when, where and so forth. Framing the problem in such a way implicitly assumes that there is an us and a them, an inside and an outside. Whether one starts with the reality of nation-states and political borders or from other types of idealised beginnings clearly affects the theorising about ethical obligations to human beings who are near versus those who are distant (see chapter by Brown for a critical analysis of statist priority views). The capabilities approach challenges this sort of formulation of the problem of global justice. And it stands in stark contrast to many other justice theories in that it conceives justice as something that can exist outside of political relationships. In Nussbaum's case, every human being, wherever we find them, has pre-political entitlements arising out of their human dignity that their own society as well as other societies must respect. However, she allocates the duties to secure capabilities domestically and internationally to institutions including domestic 'basic structures', multinational corporations, multi-lateral agencies and non-governmental organisations (Nussbaum 2006: 306–24). For Sen, justice resides not in institutions but in individuals and their capabilities (Sen 2009). Such a stance is very distinct from the common understanding that justice is the first virtue of social institutions or realised by institutions created by individuals who stand in some sort of political relation to each other.

As the capabilities approach conceives justice as residing in capabilities of individuals and as pre-political, it has global scope from the start. The global dimensions of the moral entitlement to the capability to be healthy begin right from initial recognition that every human being has a claim to basic capabilities. Because the capabilities approach eschews a fictitious social contract, and relies on free-standing philosophical and ethical reasoning, the capabilities approach has little difficulty recognising the injustice in the lives of human beings, wherever we find them. Once it is recognised that every human being has entitlements to basic capabilities, then the actions of individuals and social structures from the local to the global can be judged to be good or bad in relation to the capabilities. We can also identify the relevant obligations of different actors in relation to capabilities.

To that end, Thomas Pogge provides a helpful taxonomy of obligations (Pogge 2005a). He identifies negative duties to not harm, intermediate duties to avert harm that one's past conduct may cause in the future, and positive duties. In those situations where there is no agent of harm or immediately able to fulfil the positive duty, Sen identifies an obligation of anyone with 'effective power' to help. The possession of the capability to assist someone who has constrained basic capabilities in itself produces an obligation at least to consider helping (Sen 2009: 205–7). This may entail a person, group or institution taking a broad range of actions to help ensure the basic capabilities of human beings, wherever we find them. The importance of the 'effective power' argument is that it greatly extends the moral motivation behind the duty to rescue beyond the immediate situation of peril to the improvement of well-being while also diminishing the moral importance of national borders. It also contests the necessity of a global superstructure capable of force, as some think is necessary for global justice (Nagel 2005).

There is a danger of course that with its emphatic focus on capabilities, the capabilities approach could be interpreted as making no moral distinction between the obligations to ensure capabilities of one's own family members, of co-nationals and anyone else in the world. That would be an incorrect and narrow understanding of the capabilities approach. The capabilities approach does not focus exclusively either on establishing a fair procedure or on the end-state distribution of discreet outcomes in terms of capabilities. Rather, the capabilities approach's reasoning about addressing domestic and global health inequalities involves ethical evaluation, as part of robust public reasoning, of multiple dimensions including the causes, consequences, social distribution, persistence through generations, burdens on care-givers, possible responses as well as the relevant agents, relationships between people, and processes. The concept of capabilities is a central part of the capabilities approach's conception of justice, but not the totality of its conception. Aspects such as agency, process and power also matter for realising justice.

4. CONCLUSION

I will not try to summarise the different parts of the previous discussion but instead conclude by restating that the main aim of this chapter was to provide an introductory overview of how the capabilities approach relates to discussions on health equity, equality and justice, and global justice. From a capabilities approach perspective, health (outcome) inequalities whether nationally or globally reflect inequalities in the capabilities to be healthy. Evaluating the state of people's capabilities to be healthy – their causes, constraints, levels, distribution patterns, differential experiences, possible remedies for constraints or potential improvements – will tell us a great deal about the justness of social arrangements. This is because people's health or clinical 'health outcomes' and their antecedent capabilities to be healthy are significantly socially produced (that is, nurtured, protected, restored, neglected or thwarted) by a range of political, economic, legal, cultural and religious institutions and processes operating locally, nationally and globally. Health and longevity are significantly influenced by the physical and social environments – as well as the determinants of these environments – where human beings are born, live, work, play and age (Sen 1993: Sen 1995; Commission on Social Determinants of Health 2008; Robert Wood Johnson Foundation Commission to Build a Healthier America 2009).

At the same time, through grounding a claim to health capability in the fundamental values of liberty and equality, it becomes possible to assert that, all things considered, a government and society which allows its citizens to die prematurely or suffer impairments when they are preventable reflects a lack of concern for basic capabilities or freedoms, and does not show equal concern and respect. A well-ordered national and global society would ensure that all individuals have the capability to be healthy and at a level that is commensurate with equal human dignity in the modern world, which is their right. Rather than living in institutions, whether ideal, real or yet to exist, justice and injustice lie in the capabilities of human beings, wherever we find them. The stark inequalities and low levels of health and longevity of human beings within and across societies evidences the levels of constrained capabilities and, thus, the scale of injustice in the world.

Part 2

Who is Responsible for Remedying Global Health Inequality?

Chapter 5

RE-EXAMINING THE ETHICAL FOUNDATIONS: BEHIND THE DISTRIBUTION OF GLOBAL HEALTH

Garrett Wallace Brown

Do we have ethical obligations to promote global health equity? If so, what prioritised values should represent the satisfaction of those moral duties? These are not easy questions to answer and despite a general agreement that current inequalities in global health provision exist, as well as some agreement that a response is required, there is little consensus about what ethical foundations apply when responding to these inequalities. In an effort to provide some response to this lacuna, the purpose of this chapter is to explore three diverse normative arguments about why we might have global health responsibilities and to examine their relationship with distributive principles for the alleviation of global health inequalities. Through this examination it will be argued that current theorising about global health rests on opposing ontological worldviews about what global health should prioritise and that these pre-suppositions result in distinctively antagonistic normative demands about how we *should* calculate the distribution of global health. Moreover, by examining these ethical positions together (assuming that some movement toward the elevation of global health inequality is important) the philosophical attractiveness of a cosmopolitan approach to global health will be stressed.[1]

THINKING ETHICALLY ABOUT GLOBAL HEALTH AND GLOBAL JUSTICE

Debates about global health are full of statements about what we *should* do. These statements are usually based on two inter-related methods of normative theorising. The first method seeks to examine how current practices meet with established norms and posits a demand that humanitarian actors ought to abide by international laws, norms and standards. For example, if you were to ask the health practitioner about what normative principles should underwrite global health policy they would most likely quote various statements entrenched within global health documents, citing particular norms regarding the use of certain treatment programmes such as DOTS, or would cite policy norms related to specific global health initiatives. In this case, the judgement about what we normatively should do is based on complying with a set of common social, scientific and legal norms. As stated above, this represents one component of normative theorising, in that it seeks to make normative judgements about what we ought to do by locating the ways in which individuals and societies already define that which they consider appropriate and how certain social practices can be seen to be in accordance with these standards.

A second method seeks to make further evaluations and prescriptions about how things *should* or *ought to* be. For example, if you were to ask most political philosophers about what normative principles should underwrite the distribution of global health, they would most likely suggest that this determination requires a deeper examination than simply locating common practice or with citing existing value judgements and institutional prescriptions about what ought to happen. For them, what is of primary importance when engaging in normative theorising is to understand how these value judgements are formulated, what internal aspects and pre-suppositions underwrite the process about what we believe to be 'right' or 'wrong', and how these prioritised values relate to more idealised considerations of ethical behaviour. In this regard, this second component of normative theorising seeks to critically assess how we come to determine the rightness or wrongness of a certain behaviour or judgement, what ontological and epistemological pre-suppositions are employed during this process, and how these values rightly or wrongly underwrite the normative prescriptions about what we should do. Through this process of critical reflection the normative theorist seeks to make judgements about these value judgements themselves, and to make explicit the processes and foundational principles used to determine questions of distributive justice. In other words, the key to this kind of normative theorising is to unpack what ontological worldviews, value judgements, epistemologies and prioritisations justify the internal aspects behind the norm itself and to determine whether or not this norm and its set of justifications can be coherently and consistently defended (in both theory and by practice).

In the spirit of exposing underlying pre-suppositions involved with current global health, the central tenet of this chapter stipulates that how we institute the distribution of global health is determined almost exclusively by how ontological frames are delineated, for these frames will shape the interpretation of what ought to be prioritised. To provide a definition, ontology refers to the theory of being and existence, with reference to the contours that we see (or think we see) in the nature of things. In this regard, the determination of whether or not a normative theory actually corresponds to a present 'reality' is usually conducted with regard to a pre-supposed ontological frame which helps to order what entities exist or can be said to exist, and how otherwise disparate empirical experiences can be grounded into a hierarchy of being. To put this differently, ontologies are explicit formal specifications of how to represent the objects, concepts and entities of experience to essential qualities and relationships that hold among them. Therefore, if we are to understand how to distribute global health (or how we currently distribute global health), or how to reduce inequalities, then it is crucial to understand the common ontological frames to which these questions are usually organised and how these frames guide the normative process.

In light of this, the question that often remains unasked in global health relates to why we should do anything about global health in the first place and what underwriting pre-suppositions drive these normative assumptions. It is with exploring three normatively distinct arguments about why we should (or should not) have global health responsibilities that the rest of this chapter is dedicated. By doing so, it will be possible to expose the idiosyncratic ontologies involved in each approach as well as to provide a critical platform from which to analyse how well these approaches answer the three demands of any normative theory in relation to the distribution of global health: explanation (why), judgement (what) and prescription (who). It is through this process of comparative investigation that the philosophical attractiveness of a cosmopolitan approach to global health will be stressed.

PROXIMITY AND THE DISTRIBUTION OF GLOBAL HEALTH

We often hear the complaint that 'money is wasted on foreign aid at a time when there are plenty of people at home who require assistance'.

Underwriting this statement is what is called the *proximity thesis*. According to this thesis, people will feel stronger identification relationships to those who are nearest in communal proximity, and as a result will prioritise their distributive obligations in relation to the immediacy of these relationships.[2] The argument from proximity does not exclude the possibility that we have some obligations to those abroad, but it does stipulate that these duties will not constitute the same level of 'special obligation' that exists between family members, neighbours, co-nationals and fellow citizens. The proximity thesis is presented as a foundational empirical condition of identity and social enculturation, in which normative determinations about distributive justice will correspond to claims of existing solidarities and the intensity of obligation conditioned by the immediate proximity of those relationships.

If we accept the empirical claim regarding proximity as correct, as many social justice theorists do, then it is possible to generate key normative arguments for why we should favour special obligations between co-nationals as taking precedence over other individuals beyond our borders. As David Miller argues, national and communal sentiments are important and necessary conditions in establishing the motivations for, and the reciprocal conditions of, social justice (Miller 1999). To ignore the meaningfulness of these special obligations on our social lives would negate an important aspect of our human condition and the conditions on which social justice rests. Although we should have some responsibilities to others beyond communal borders based on general humanitarian concerns, these responsibilities should remain a secondary 'sub-duty' and special duties to co-nationals should take precedence over other international obligations (Miller 2007). In regard to how this may play out in relation to global health, Miller presents the following case:

> Suppose that a flu pandemic breaks out and the government only has sufficient vaccine to inoculate a limited number of vulnerable people against the disease. It does not seem wrong in this case to give priority to treating compatriots, that is to supply the vaccine to all those fellow-citizens identified by age or other relevant criteria as belonging to the vulnerable group, before sending any surplus abroad, even though it is reasonable to assume that some foreigners will be more vulnerable to the flu than some compatriots selected for vaccination. And this remains true even if we know

that those more vulnerable foreigners will not receive the vaccine from their own health services. (Miller 2007: 45)

In making this determination, Miller suggests that the context of 'social justice' is different from normal appeals about justice, since 'social justice is practised among people who are citizens of the same political community' and 'our thinking about justice should be conditioned by existing empirical realities' (Miller 2007: 16).[3] As a result, 'the idea of justice is contextually determined' and 'we need to ask whether the institutions and modes of human association that we find within nation-states, and which form the context within which ideas of social justice are developed and applied, are also to be found at the international level, and if not, how we should understand human relationships across national borders' (Miller 2007: 14). In doing so, however, it is clear from Miller that proximity and relational duties are what matter in the formulation of just responsibilities and that when calculating the distribution of global health, we should not be afraid to appeal to our co-national 'ethical intuitions' (Miller 2007: 45).

In unpacking these arguments it is important to highlight that a specific ontological frame underpins the claims of Miller and other like-minded scholars. In essence, this ontology asserts that globalisation and its transnational spaces do not represent a form of *relational* interdependency to a point where it resembles conditions of social co-operation and economic institutionalism as found within the nation-state. In this regard, the current global order and its transnational structure does not (and possibly cannot) represent the basic institutional conditions analogous to the conditions under which many traditional political theorists argue justice should/can apply. In this case, the argument about the scope of justice rests on an empirical assessment about whether or not there is enough of an identification relationship between peoples at the global level to motivate duties of justice and whether transnational spaces are actually creating a sense of cosmopolitan identity (Cabrera 2010) or promoting cultural distinctiveness and renewed national sentiments (Saul 2005). In other words, the debate about global justice involves evaluations about current solidarities regarding universal humanity, our identification with this common humanity, and whether these new transnational identities are strong enough to provide a *global horizon* for duties of global justice (Vertovec and Cohen 2002). As implied above, a common critique of

the existence of a global horizon is that globalisation and its trans-
formational aspects have been 'exaggerated' by more cosmopolitan-
minded scholars and that there are still justified arguments for national
prioritisations when determining the boundaries of justice and political
membership (Kymlicka 2011).

The political manifestations of these sorts of arguments are evident
within many current debates about global health. Perhaps most
notably, this underwriting logic underpins what is often called the
statist approach. As Sarah Davies suggests, 'according to the statist perspective . . . the health of individuals requires effective state structures
. . . [and] although this perspective recognises the need for multilateral
responses to some health crises, its central premise remains on secur-
ing the state' (Davies 2010: 21). From this, 'the statist perspective holds
that health issues must be addressed when they directly impact the
economic, political and military security of the state' (Davies 2010: 14).
Like the proximity thesis above, the argument is not that we have no
obligations to others at the global level, but that the prioritisation of
those duties relates specifically to the state as the referent object and to
the prioritised interests of that political community.

Since the referent object within this ontology is the state and its
security, it engenders particular normative conclusions in relation to
global health responsibility. The basic premise is that because global
health not only impacts on the security of the state, but also because it
can impact on the stability of the state system as a whole, states should
have responsibilities toward alleviating potential threats to the state
(Price-Smith 2009). This is not only in regard to safeguarding the internal institutions required for domestic justice (Garrett 2001), as Thomas
Nagel would argue is crucial for a system of justice (Nagel 2005), but
also in regard to pursuing international efforts to respond to key threats
to national security (Fidler 1999). Nevertheless, to be clear, because
of the overriding importance of state security, when determining the
appropriation of global health inequalities, the distribution should by
necessity prioritise the security needs of the state first as well as frame
all ethical considerations in relation to this prioritised demand.

Adherence to this position results in several idiosyncratic political
formations and distributional modes in relation to global health. First,
because national interests are prioritised, there is a tendency to engage
in the *securitisation* of global health and to think narrowly of international efforts as representing a form of *microbialpolitik* (Fidler 1999:

19). As a result, there is a propensity to give a prioritised focus to the securitisation of transborder infectious diseases while ignoring other health-related emergencies. Although there are arguments to suggest that states are more willing to give increased resources when issues are framed in terms of security, it is also the case that security prioritisation means that these resources remain narrowly targeted (McInnes and Lee 2006). One consequence of this is that normative appeals to security become most suitable for addressing acute crises, but often remain inadequate for addressing the underlying causes of infectious diseases, be they political, economic, social or cultural (Youde 2005).

Second, addressing global health from a statist perspective can lead to what Wimmer and Glick-Schiller have described as 'methodological nationalism' and an uncritical acceptance that current state boundaries correspond neatly with national boundaries and that these boundaries represent the only institutional scope available for constructing a sense of citizenship and political obligation (Wimmer and Glick-Schiller 2002: 304). The problem is that by remaining anchored to existing political boundaries as delimiting the possible scope of justice and effective collective action, it can blindly overlook more appropriate and effective forms of political and social organisation that could/should exist between states and beyond (Orbinski 2007). This problem is highlighted particularly well within the statist logic itself, which acknowledges a paradoxical situation where states represent the agents of prioritised interests while at the same time recognising that many health threats are transborder phenomena which cannot be addressed by a single state actor or a collection of states. This suggests that there is scope for more cosmopolitan-inspired schemes of global governance, but because of ontological framing these are dismissed as only secondary components to the preferred position of state-based multilateralism.

Third, as Susan Peterson (2006) and Simon Rushton (2011) have suggested, if the normative argument about global health is framed solely in terms of security then most Western countries will not face the same threats as most of the world's population and they will therefore dedicate insufficient resources to those most in need (as Miller's 'ethical intuition' suggested). Since this distribution can be rationalised within the statist ontology, it will assist in 'relieving Westerners of any moral obligation to respond to health crises beyond their own national borders' (Peterson 2006: 46). This is because if security is the overall specification of how to represent the objects and concepts of study within an overarching hierarchical relationship of existence, as this ontology suggests, then any normative prescriptions about distributive justice would need to correspond with this overarching worldview.

LIFEBOAT ETHICS AND THE DISTRIBUTION OF GLOBAL HEALTH

At a recent dinner party a guest made the suggestion that a global justice approach to global health failed to capture the 'natural fact' that 'diseases are part of a natural process to remove excessive overpopulation and restore natural balance'. From this initial position, the dinner guest wondered if it *should* always be considered a bad thing when people die of preventable diseases.

In thinking about how one could respond to the guest's question it is necessary to unpack the logic that underwrites the concern about the maintenance of 'natural order' and to come up with suggestions for why, given this logic, one might still have some level of global health responsibility and to determine what this would normatively demand. In thinking about this it becomes clear that the guest's argument is grounded in the tradition broadly associated with *Malthusianism* and its philosophical offspring, *lifeboat ethics*. When unpacking this argument it is possible to see the guest's logic developing as follows. First, the statement is based on an ontology which suggests that nature seeks a symbiotic equilibrium and through a process of natural selection nature will 'thin out' weaker organisms in favour of stronger organisms. In terms of normative reflection, this categorisation acts as the essential quality and empirical frame from which normative theorising must engage as well as satisfy. Second, the argument is supported by a further empirical assertion that the earth is made up of various groups that act like natural organisms and each group contains inherent social characteristics that will allow it to adapt or not adapt to processes of natural selection. Third, since the world is a global sphere of limited resources and finite capacities, a zero sum condition of group survival is inevitable. Fourth, given this logic, the measurement of whether a 'civilisational organism' is successful in adapting depends solely on its ability to survive these 'natural processes' and therefore we should judge the worthiness of a group by its capacity to survive various natural 'corrections' toward equilibrium.

Assuming the ontological and empirical validity of this logic, which in my opinion is questionable, it is possible for the lifeboat ethicist to posit four normative conclusions in relation to why one should still have a level of global health responsibility. Furthermore, from this natural logic it is possible to generate a general normative direction about what should be prioritised within this distribution and for whom. The first normative conclusion is that stronger groups or civilisations should pursue selected global health initiatives in order to survive processes of natural equilibrium and to pre-empt external threats that pose potential danger. From this, given an assumed condition of limited resources and natural capacities, stronger civilisations should prioritise themselves because natural equilibrium represents a 'lifeboat' that should not be overburdened by providing high levels of survival assistance to weaker groups. As it was suggested by the dinner guest, diseases are viewed as 'part of a natural process' to counter overpopulation and to establish a symbiotic natural equilibrium. Because of this, it is in humankind's overall best interest to 'let these natural processes run their course'. In terms of ethics and morals, since natural selection is an 'instrument of natural order' the decision to prioritise stronger civilisations and to allow weaker groups to perish naturally is consistent with this natural logic and it therefore does not represent an immoral stance, but pertains to amoral empirical necessity regarding the survival of superior civilisations and the conditions for human survival as a whole. As a result, strong civilisations should pursue global health initiatives that seek to prioritise the survival of their civilisation by containing and suppressing external threats. Since certain issues of global health represent possible threats to the 'lifeboat', those within it should dedicate sufficient civilisational resources toward stemming the most immediate and clear threats, like the spread of transborder infectious diseases (Hardin 1974b).

The implications in terms of the distribution of global health relate strictly to consequentialist calculations regarding containment and civilisational survival. In this regard, as with the statist approach outlined in the prior section, the normative focus for a lifeboat ethic relates specifically to maintaining the security of one group over another. Although statism speaks in terms of state security in relation to global health, whereas a lifeboat ethic utilises the language of social evolution and survival, in both theories the distribution of goods and services within global health is determined by appeals to the security of specific communities and the hierarchical prioritisation of certain groups over others. Furthermore, although the lifeboat metaphor is presented as an ethical position, in that it seeks to determine what is good or bad and what the basis of that calculation is, it is nonetheless portrayed as representing an amoral condition of *necessity* and nature, in which human beings are absolved of moral culpability (but not necessarily of moral remorse), since to do otherwise would result in a 'tragedy of the commons' that would ultimately threaten the entire human species and run counter to the evolutionary laws of nature (Hardin 1968).

Assuming the correctness of the lifeboat metaphor and the ontology that underpins it, some normative justifications for the distribution of health can be rendered tenable. This is because, if survival toward equilibrium is the overall specification of how to represent the objects and concepts of study within an overarching hierarchical relationship of being, as this ontology does, then any normative command must mirror and satisfy the conditions of this overarching relationship. To do otherwise, according to lifeboat ethics, is to contradict 'reality' and our understanding of the world. If avoiding this requires the favouritism of some more advanced and adaptable groups over others, even at the demise of these other groups, then we should do so, since this action accords with the ontological pre-suppositions of necessity. As Garrett Hardin argues, 'our survival demands that we govern our actions by the ethics of a lifeboat, harsh though they may be . . . for posterity will be satisfied with nothing less' (Hardin 1974a).

In thinking about why we might want to be sceptical about a lifeboat ethic, it is important to re-examine and challenge its key ontological foundations and the way the lifeboat ethicist frames their empirical and normative logic. First, it is important to note that this position rests on a problematic teleology that frames all human experiences as being related to a pre-determined natural purpose or 'posterity'. It also seemingly assumes, quite incorrectly, that nature will deliver a natural equilibrium that is cognitively comprehensible and that it will always accommodate the survival of certain superior organisms. This claim is made despite the fact that it is epistemologically uncertain what a definition of 'superior' actually entails prior to future outcomes. Like many critiques of strict consequentialism, these kinds of calculations can be troublesome in the face of methodological issues regarding epistemic uncertainty and the inability to know how the results will pan out prior to the action taken. In opposition, the assumption of an accommodating natural equilibrium may very well not be the case empirically or consequently, for under its own logic, a reliance on natural order must also then include the possible extinction of the entire human species. This may come as a result of our own industrial cleverness, or result from something outside the biosphere like a large meteorite strike.

Second, there is a tendency for the lifeboat ethicist to frame moral activity as also being part of a natural process and to justify all actions in relation to an ontologically pre-supposed natural order. This *a priori* ontological position then acts as the sole criterion from which to measure, judge and normatively respond to all human activities. By doing so, it renders a deterministic vision of human experience and removes moral agency as a potential process of natural order. In other words, by suggesting the existence of a teleological purpose of nature, which is inherently amoral, it renders a deterministic vision of human nature and removes the prospects of moral agency as playing an important role as part of natural order itself. By denying a role for morality in the natural order, what is normatively permissible can include more than just 'letting nature run its course' through acts of ethical omission, for under this logic it could also be used to justify more direct survival strategies which may include appeals to eugenics or other 'necessary' means to keep the lifeboat afloat.

Third, like the statist position, the lifeboat ethicist assumes that every human belongs to one particular identifiable group and that these groups are static entities with delineated borders and inherent natural capacities. However, by doing so the lifeboat ethicist commits two key fallacies: a) he does not account for the role of luck in determining how a group's natural capacities are developed; and b) he does not account for the fact that in many cases the causes of misfortune are not strictly 'natural', but are often caused explicitly by the reasoned actions of human beings.

COSMOPOLITANISM AND THE DISTRIBUTION OF GLOBAL HEALTH

A few months ago I attended a rally being held on my campus to raise awareness about the destruction caused by HIV/AIDS in Africa. During this rally a woman with a megaphone yelled slogans along the lines that 'we should view all human beings as equally valuable, that everyone shares certain basic human rights to healthcare and that we *must* take our global responsibilities to those affected by HIV/AIDS more seriously'. In thinking about how to ground this statement, it is clear that the student is appealing to the deontological view that all human beings have an equal worth and that our ethical decisions about distributive justice and global health should accord with a universalised category that can act as a litmus test for whether or not a particular distribution is viewed as morally permissible. Contrary to the consequentialism of lifeboat ethics, where a utility calculus only considers how to maximise a particular value as universally as possible, a deontological approach examines whether this act would violate a universal duty to humanity itself, regardless of what overall consequence will result (Donagan 1977).

The grounding for the student's more cosmopolitan approach to global health is most likely determined by three inter-related arguments. First, cosmopolitans argue that any scheme of global health based on the proximity thesis is morally arbitrary when it formulates its distributive principles. This is because it is simply a matter of happenstance whether a person is born in one place versus another. In other words, being born into one set of institutional relationships (that is, a civilisation or a state) is not a matter of moral choice by the individual who is born into that relationship. In fact, where a person is born is purely a matter of luck and, as many cosmopolitans argue, it is morally suspect to determine what a person is entitled to solely on the good fortune of birth alone. As a result, many cosmopolitans have argued that the requirement of communal membership as an over-riding precondition for determining the scope of justice is unconvincing and thus weakens the normative appeal of the statist position (Caney 2005).

When placed in comparison to the ontological frames of the proximity thesis and lifeboat ethics, the cosmopolitan argues that these pre-suppositions conflate luck with duty and as a result fail to appreciate the universal characteristic of human morality and dignity. As a contrasting theory, most cosmopolitans argue that it is important to prioritise human moral worth as a universally 'protected value' because this value captures what is distinctively human in our nature. For the cosmopolitan, it is imperative to consider ethical decisions in relation to whether the moral duty can also be conceived as universally valid. Otherwise, the idea of human morality no longer represents a self-imposed law onto oneself, but rather, like the earlier critique of lifeboat ethics, becomes a deterministic act of coercion outside the realm of moral agency. Because of this, many cosmopolitans invoke Kant's *categorical imperative* when considering the conditions of justice, and uphold the idea that we should 'act in such a way that you treat humanity, whether in your own person or in the person of another, always at the same time as an end, and never as a means' (Kant 1981: 36). In practice, these metaphysical principles have provided the inspirational ground for appeals to the protection of *universal human rights* (Pogge 2002) to the fulfilment of human *capabilities* (Nussbaum 2005),[4] to the primacy of *human security* (Booth 2007) and to the establishment of mutually consistent maxims of universal public right.

Second, a cosmopolitan approach broadens the contextual conceptualisation involved with relational theories of justice and by doing so seeks to undermine distributions that are strictly based on the proximity thesis. This logic suggests that if John Rawls was right to claim that justice is the first principle of any scheme of social co-operation, and that globalisation has 'stretched' the need for co-operative relationships beyond the state, then the scope of justice should also extend beyond the borders of states. As several cosmopolitans have argued, international economic interdependency has come to resemble something like the conditions of social co-operation and 'basic institutions' that originally motivated Rawls' domestic concern for distributive justice (Beitz 1992). As Charles Beitz argues, under Rawls' own logic, 'if evidence of global economic and political interdependence shows the existence of a global scheme of social cooperation, we should not view national boundaries as having fundamental moral significance' (Beitz 1979: 376). As Brian Barry furthers, this form of impartial moral cosmopolitanism 'shows itself to be distinctive in its denial that membership of a society is of deep moral significance when the claims that people can legitimately make on one another are addressed' (Barry 1998: 145). This is because cosmopolitanism morally demands that 'human beings are in some fundamental sense equal' and that to satisfy this moral principle would require further principles of impartial justice that 'others could not reasonably reject' (Barry 1998: 146). As with the case against lifeboat ethics, this demands that we privilege the 'right' over the 'good' and that the determination of what is 'right' requires an adherence to universal principles of impartial justice and deliberation that no one could reasonably reject.

As stated before, one primary component of the statist ontology is the belief that globalisation has not developed to a sufficient point of relational interdependence where debates about justice are held to apply. As was outlined earlier, in relation to global health, theorists like Miller suggested that special duties to co-nationals should take precedence over other international obligations. In outlining his argument, Miller used an example of flu inoculations to illustrate how this prioritisation to co-nations morally corresponds with our 'ethical intuitions'. A key aspect of Miller's justification is that whereas co-nationals are embroiled in a relational system of social justice, this relational element is not evident at the global level. As a result, when determining who gets what and why, Miller suggests that 'our thinking about justice should be conditioned by existing empirical realities' (Miller 2007: 16).

Nevertheless, if this logic is correct, we must acknowledge the increasing empirical evidence which suggests that, at a very minimum, there are causal components of interaction that exist at the global level. These interactions can be measured through locating key interdependent relationships produced by global markets, global economies, transnational spaces and cultural cross-pollinations. In terms of global health, unlike Miller's seeming assumption that each nation-state is largely self-contained and as a result 'self-responsible', there are several studies to suggest that the global economy and the existing political order have profound effects on the health and well-being of individuals across borders (Labonte et al. 2009; Brown and Labonte 2011). This has led some cosmopolitans, like Thomas Pogge, to suggest that our willing participation in the international market creates an 'interactional context', and therefore implicates those benefiting from these global interactions with a set of mitigating responsibilities – such as responsibilities for global health. As Pogge proposes, there are injustices involved within the current interactional structure and that this institutional architecture systematically violates the basic human rights of certain populations. Since the minimum demands of justice command that we do not violate the negative rights of others, and if one's involvement in the international structure systematically supports a violation of these rights, then there is 'causal material involvement' and we are morally responsible to reform the system (Pogge 2004: 134–7).

Third, cosmopolitans often suggest that statist ontologies overly fetishise the status quo, which, although capturing some aspects of existing political solidarity, tends to lock in existing political communities as static entities. Cosmopolitans counter this by suggesting that the nation-state is simply a political construction that does not contain – in and of itself – an inherent moral worth. As some cosmopolitans argue, the state is nothing more than the product of human invention and ingenuity, and it is not a static entity that needs to be intrinsically protected from new forms of moral and political alteration. In this regard, the state is something that can be reconstructed, reformulated and, consequently, transformed into something else (Beck 2006). If this is true, as cosmopolitanism specifies, then the state is merely a constructed institutional entity designed to co-ordinate the political relationships between people. If globalisation has broadened the scope of those relationships beyond state borders, as even a statist position on global health admits, then the state loses its bounded saliency and relevance in favour of new political formulations that can better capture the inter-relations that exist in a globalised world (Held and McGrew 2007).

Although the cosmopolitan approach does not provide a clear blueprint about how to move from cosmopolitan theory to cosmopolitical practice, it can nevertheless highlight particular ethical shortcomings that exist within the current state system, and these are often presented as moral foundations for global reform. And it is here, in thinking about how to reform the global system, where new and innovative research is required not only to create stronger links between global empirical experience and institutional responsibilities, but also to help capture more succinctly the ways in which our everyday lives are interlocked with expanding transnational spaces, global experiences and the political implications that result from an increasingly globalised world. For the cosmopolitan argues that it is only through challenging existing ontological pre-suppositions regarding borders, security and the survival of the fittest that we can hope to come to terms with the inequities of contemporary global health and beyond.

CONCLUSION

This chapter began by asking whether we have ethical obligations to promote global health and, if so, what prioritised values should represent the satisfaction of these ethical demands. In order to assess some key ways in which we make determinations concerning the distribution of global health, this chapter has explored three alternative normative arguments about why we should have some level of global health responsibility and how corresponding distributive principles regarding global health prioritisations are framed. In doing so, it has been argued that many prescriptions for how to institute the distribution of health are pre-determined by how ontological frames are delineated, for these frames critically shape the interpretation of what ought to be prioritised.

In two of the cases explored – proximity/statist and lifeboat ethics – there was a prioritisation of some people over others. It was only in relation to the deontological cosmopolitan position that the permissibility of excluding some for the benefit of others was deemed unethical as a matter of right. Although the examination provided in this chapter is rudimentary and only touches the surface of what is involved within these debates, it does nevertheless render an interesting image. Namely, when we think about global health and responsibility, and if we truly wish to change these prioritisations toward a more equitable relationship at the global level, then it will require more universally consistent normative prescriptions about distributive justice. It also rendered another interesting normative conclusion: at the moment, given the philosophical options available, and given the increasing disparity between the richest and the poorest, the healthy and the ill – and if we believe reaching a better level of global health equity to be a morally important endeavour – then how we frame this response will by necessity have to respond to the challenges posed by cosmopolitanism. The question to ask, and to which we should be engaged with in debates about global health, is whether we feel that the ontologically determined trade-offs involved with the proximity thesis and lifeboat amorality are ethically irresponsible and whether we should continue to treat their pre-suppositions as simply a matter of empirical fact and necessity. Since the current system often frames and justifies distributions in terms of these kinds of prioritisations/pre-suppositions, it is important not to forget that these models continue to generate moral remainders as represented by those believed to be outside the 'proximity' or who are purposely left out of the 'lifeboat'. And this is of ethical significance, since it should be remembered that these individuals do not suddenly disappear, but are simply excused away. And in this regard, despite the fact that these prioritisations are often presented as ethically justified by their advocates, it is important for us to remember that they are not unequivocally convincing in also claiming that they are morally just.

Notes

1. This chapter is based on an altered and augmented argument found in G. W. Brown, 'Distributing Who Gets What and Why: Four Normative Approaches to Global Health', *Global Policy*, vol .3, no. 3 (2012).
2. See Cole's contribution to this volume for a discussion of one example of the proximity argument in healthcare policy in the UK.
3. See Cole's chapter for an argument that argues for including rather than excluding illegal migrants among those who are entitled to this bounded social justice.
4. See Venkatapuram's chapter for an expanded argument using a capabilities approach to global health justice.

Chapter 6

GLOBAL HEALTH AND RESPONSIBILITY

Gillian Brock

1. INTRODUCTION

A striking feature concerning the state of global health is that it is characterised by some radical disparities, including those in life expectancy, maternal mortality and malaria-related deaths. Do we have any responsibilities with respect to improving global health? I begin my answer to this question by surveying a number of international practices that contribute to poor global health. We can then appreciate the wide range of different kinds of international practices and policies that facilitate poor global health. Which, if any, are we obligated to reform in our decidedly non-ideal world? How should we allocate responsibilities fairly in bringing about some necessary reforms? I argue that there is an important class of remedial responsibilities that falls on many citizens of affluent, developed states, and their primary agents of change, governments. In order to appreciate why this conclusion follows, I analyse the notion of remedial responsibilities and the grounds on which it may fairly be allocated.

2. GLOBAL HEALTH: SOME PROBLEMS AND PATTERNS

One of the most striking features about the state of global health is that it is characterised by radical inequalities. Here is just a sample of the more widely noticed kinds. Life expectancy at birth varies enormously: life expectancy in Sierra Leone or Afghanistan is about forty years, whereas those lucky enough to be born in Japan or Australia enjoy a life expectancy of twice that at approximately eighty (Benatar and Upshur 2011: 14–15). Similarly, there is huge variation in maternal mortality: a Canadian woman's lifetime risk of dying from childbirth or pregnancy complications is 1 in 11,000, whereas for a woman in the Niger it is 1 in 7 (Labonte and Schrecker 2011: 24–36). Whereas malaria is almost entirely absent in high-income countries, it kills around a million people per year elsewhere (United Nations 2009).

A largely accurate explanation for these types of differences involves poverty and material deprivation (Labonte and Schrecker 2011: 24–36). Undernourishment, slum dwelling conditions, lack of access to clean water, excessive smoke from cooking fires, and lack of resources for adequate healthcare can all contribute to poor health outcomes. However, we should resist the inference that greater wealth will automatically deliver better health, and that policies that promote economic growth are therefore the best way to achieve good population health. There is a threshold level (at about US$5,000) beyond which the relationship between life expectancy at birth and per capita incomes is inconclusive: indeed, we see many countries with low per capita incomes with very good life expectancies at birth (Labonte and Schrecker 2011: 27; Birn 2011: 43). Costa Rica is one well-known example: though per capita income in Costa Rica is about $10,500 per year, life expectancy is seventy-nine, notably more than the seventy-eight years those who reside in the US can expect to live, where per capita income is greater than $45,000 (Labonte and Schrecker 2011: 28). And Cuba presents an even more striking case (Birn 2011: 37). Material prosperity has a role to play, but social, political and economic decisions play a far greater one. Indeed, social changes can have significant consequences for health. Two examples are rapid increases in urbanisation (which can affect diet, for instance) or globalisation, which has allowed the consolidation of power over food systems, which can also lead to consumption patterns deleterious to health.

The distribution of power and of social, political and economic resources is crucial in influencing and explaining population health (Birn 2011). Understanding these ideas requires an analysis of the social determinants of health: factors that shape health at various levels including the household, community, national and global levels. Living conditions both at the household and community level can cause numerous ailments including respiratory, gastrointestinal or metabolic diseases (Birn 2011: 39–42). Availability of potable water and adequate sanitation are key factors. Though water is essential for life, more than a billion people (or one-sixth of the world's population) have an inadequate supply (Birn 2011: 40). The facts about access to adequate sanitation are even more striking – almost half the world's population has inadequate access to basic sanitation facilities, which can result in soil contamination and increased rates of communicable diseases (Birn 2011: 40). Other key factors include nutrition and food security (over 50 per cent of child deaths are attributable to poor nutrition), housing conditions, public health and healthcare services, and transportation (Birn 2011: 40–5). Social policies and government regulation (or lack thereof) can also affect health in dramatic ways, including in the domains of education, taxation, labour and environmental regulations. Patterns of unequal resource distribution and political power play a fundamental role in the social determinants of health, so in effectively addressing radical health inequalities we cannot ignore these other more basic factors (Birn 2011: 40–5).

Furthermore, the poor and marginalised suffer disproportionately from a range of health problems and will feel the effects of others more greatly. Historically, infectious diseases have caused more morbidity and mortality than any other cause including wars (Selgelid 2011: 89). Tuberculosis alone has killed a billion people during the last two centuries (Selgelid 2011: 89). But infectious diseases do not affect us all equally. Infectious diseases primarily affect the poor and marginalised who are more likely to live in the kinds of crowded and poor conditions conducive to spreading infectious diseases, be malnourished which also weakens immune systems, lack adequate hygiene provisions necessary to prevent or treat diseases, or lack access to adequate healthcare should they become infected (Selgelid 2005: 272–89; Selgelid 2011). Infectious diseases therefore cause more morbidity and mortality in developing countries than they do in developed countries. However, the vulnerability of the poor or marginalised to disease should be of concern to all of us, since epidemics in one country can easily spread to others (and become more virulent and harder to treat in the process). At least in such cases, rich countries have good, self-interested reasons to care about healthcare improvement and poverty reduction in developing countries, in order to protect their own populations adequately. Yet, such global public good type arguments are in fact quite limited and do not generalise to a range of other poor health conditions.[1]

Is all health inequality morally troublesome? We might tend to think it must be, but on reflection we see that matters are not straightforward here. For example, some important differences between male and female patterns of health and illness – indeed, life expectancy itself –

suggest there might be some inequalities that it would be very difficult, if not impossible, to eliminate (Payne 2006; Doyal and Payne 2011: 5–62; Birn 2011: 47). International health inequalities are very often rightly disturbing, such as those concerning the differences in child mortality before age five or mothers' death rates during labour. What is troubling in such cases is that the disparity shows such problems are tractable – we have the means radically to reduce (say) child deaths under age five. Is it fair that some should suffer so greatly when others do not? Is it not unjust that there should be such clear losers in the 'natural lottery', constituted by where one happens to have been born? Should such an arbitrary fact determine one's life prospects in such radical ways? As Norman Daniels argues, health inequalities among social groups are unjust or unfair when they are a product of an unjust distribution in socially controllable factors that affect population health (Daniels 2008; Daniels 2011: 97–107). Many health inequalities result from international practices that harm health quite directly, such as through our failure to build worker health and safety protections into our trade agreements (Daniels 2011: 101). In such cases, since many of the causal factors that lead to poor health are socially controllable, it is in our power to remedy these. As we are therefore in a position to change global health, we must understand what we are then obligated to do. The next section begins our analysis.

3. GLOBAL HEALTH AND RESPONSIBILITIES: WHO HAS RESPONSIBILITIES CONCERNING GLOBAL HEALTH? WHAT SHOULD BE DONE?

As we have seen, the poor state of global health is widely documented. Moreover, as Thomas Pogge notes, about one-third of annual human deaths are traceable to extreme poverty (way below the $5,000 threshold previously discussed) and, moreover, are easily preventable through such measures as safe drinking water, vaccines, antibiotics, better nutrition or cheap re-hydration packs (Pogge 2008a, 2008c). Is there an obligation to prevent such deaths? Are there any duties to address global health and, if so, what arguments can be marshalled for this position?

First, what are we obligated to do to alleviate world poverty? Thomas Pogge famously argues that whatever the merits of the case that we should help more, there is much more clearly an obligation to harm less

(Pogge 2008c). How do we currently harm the poor? In multiple ways, he argues (Pogge 2008c; Pogge 2005b: 55–84). One can challenge the legitimacy of our currently highly uneven global distributive patterns concerning income and wealth, which has emerged from a single historical process pervaded by injustices (such as slavery and colonialism). One might also criticise the dense web of institutional arrangements that we fail to reform which 'foreseeably and avoidably' perpetuate poverty. Pogge has argued that the way in which we fail to reform various institutional arrangements, which foreseeably and avoidably perpetuate massive global poverty, is morally culpable. Notable among these arrangements are the international resource and borrowing privileges, which allow whomever holds power over a territory to sell the country's resources legitimately (the international resource privilege) and borrow in the country's name (the international borrowing privilege), no matter how power was obtained. These privileges have disastrous effects for developing countries, especially in fostering corrupt and oppressive governments, as they incentivise seizing power through illegitimate means and enable the consolidation of that power by providing a steady stream of resources helpful in maintaining corrupt and repressive regimes.

But these are by no means the only institutional arrangements that perpetuate poverty. The list would also include upholding grossly unjust intellectual property regimes that require all members of the World Trade Organization to grant twenty-year product patents which effectively make new medicines unaffordable for most of the world's population. Reforming these unjust trade-related intellectual property arrangements (TRIPS) is a major focus of some of Pogge's important recent work (Pogge 2011: 241–50).

Advocates of such intellectual property arrangements often argue that these patenting schemes are necessary to compensate innovators for the large investments necessary to develop new drugs. Pogge is not unaware of the need for incentives and rewards to compensate for research and development investment into new drugs, and he presents an alternative proposal which can overcome at least seven failings of the present pharmaceutical regime, which would include: high prices; neglect of diseases concentrated among the poor unable to afford the high prices for drugs (such as malaria or tuberculosis); a bias towards developing maintenance rather than curative or preventative drugs; massive wastefulness in policing patent law; the illegal manufacture of counterfeit and often ineffectual drugs; excessive marketing; and inattention to ensuring patients use the drugs in beneficial ways (Pogge 2011).

Pogge proposes a 'Health Impact Fund' (HIF) as one major component of necessary structural reform. Financed mainly by governments, this proposed global agency would present pharmaceutical innovators with the opportunity to participate, during the first ten years a drug is on the market, in the HIF's 'reward pool'; successful innovators would be entitled to a share of rewards equal to a share of the global health impact of HIF-registered products (for a discussion of how impact of drugs should be measured, see Yukiko Asada's and Nicole Hassoun's chapters). The innovators would have to make the drug widely and cheaply available wherever it was needed and, indeed, would be incentivised to do so. Pogge, and an interdisciplinary team, develop the details of the scheme, so that it presents a clear alternative to the current regime and one that is not guilty of the seven main failings identified above. Importantly, it provides significant rewards for the development of drugs that would address some of the most widespread global diseases concentrated among the poor, who currently do not have the purchasing power to capture the attention of drug developers. Since Pogge has presented a feasible alternative to TRIPS agreements for rewarding drug innovators, he argues that our imposition of these regimes on the world's poor is not only harmful but morally culpable, and our failure to reform current regimes is unjust (for an alternative mechanism by which to encourage pharmaceutical companies to focus energies on development of drugs for the poor, see Nicole Hassoun's chapter).

The idea of allocating responsibility with respect to global health in general is a complex issue. Allen Buchanan and Matthew DeCamp offer some guidelines for translating our shared obligation to 'do something' to improve global health into a more determinate set of obligations (Buchanan 2009: Chapter 10; Buchanan and DeCamp 2011: 119–28). They argue that states in particular have more extensive and specific responsibilities than is typically assumed to be the case, as the current primary agents of distributive justice, influential actors in the burden of disease, and indeed in our world, having the greatest impact on the health of individuals. But non-state actors (such as the World Trade Organization and global corporations) have important responsibilities as well. Furthermore, institutional innovation is needed to distribute responsibilities more fairly and comprehensively, and to ensure accountability.

Some of the determinate obligations they identify for states include: to avoid committing injustice that has health-harming effects, such as not to fight unjust wars abroad or assist in training military personnel of states likely to use force unjustly. In supporting unjust governments and upholding the state system, which bestows privileges such as the international and resource privileges, we contribute to upholding unjust regimes that have health-harming effects. Simply refraining from such activities could do much to improve global health. As one example, consider how from 2000 to 2006 3.9 million people died in the Congo from war. Every violent death in that war zone is accompanied by no fewer than sixty-two 'non-violent' deaths in the region, from starvation, disease and associated events. The indirect effects of war on health are often unappreciated (Buchanan and DeCamp 2011: 123).

Under our current world order, states are supposed to be the primary guarantors of their citizens' human rights. As Buchanan and DeCamp note, this arrangement can, in many cases, usefully be deployed to improve health outcomes. Though the full content of the right to health has yet to be developed, this approach can still assist in allocating duties as in many cases it is undeniable that the right has not been fulfilled for the very worst off (for attempts to account for the content of a human right to health, see Adina Preda's and Eszter Kollar's chapters). What about cases where states are unable or unwilling to act? There is much we in the international community can do to assist to secure this right for the very worst off. Setting up the Global Fund (which aims to address AIDS, tuberculosis and malaria) is one such example of effective transnational action with positive results (Buchanan and DeCamp 2011: 123).

The obligation not to contribute to or uphold unjust arrangements that have health-harming effects for which Pogge, Buchanan and DeCamp (inter alia) argue will, when more fully considered, give rise to numerous obligations in areas not traditionally strongly associated with issues of health, such as arms-trading and trade more generally, dealing with climate change, or taxation practices. I consider some of these domains next.

The link between international arms-trading and global health is easy to appreciate (Mahmudi-Azer 2011: 166–72). First, the global arms trade has an enormous socio-economic impact, but also greatly undesirable effects for human health and the environment. These adverse impacts include death, injury and maiming from weapons-use in conflict, but there is massive opportunity cost to health, economic development and human well-being when there is large-scale diversion of resources from health and human services into weapons expenditure (Mahmudi-Azer 2011: 166–8). The impact of conflict can be far-reaching and includes important effects on children, such as psychological damage, loss of educational opportunities, destruction of families and nurturing environments, abuse, and the coerced conscription of child soldiers. With trade in weapons fast growing and currently constituting the largest economy in the world, the effects on human health and well-being are worrisome (Mahmudi-Azer 2011: 166–8).

Second, health can certainly affect trade, as is the case when a global epidemic hampers trade. Furthermore, it is clear that robust interests in trade can undermine health-related priorities and practice (Koivusalo 2011: 143–54). For instance, trade liberalisation policies in agricultural products can affect price, availability and access to basic food commodities, with consequences including less healthy diets for local populations and related issues of food security (Koivusalo 2011: 143–9). Furthermore, trade liberalisation has made available more hazardous substances such as tobacco and alcohol, leading to unhealthy consumption patterns (Koivusalo 2011: 143–54). Greater centralisation of ownership and control in the agribusiness industry, greater enclosure by corporations of food sources once held in common, and diversion of food resources, particularly grain, into biofuel production can all result in critical food shortages (Gill and Bakker 2011: 221–38). Poor developing countries may be more vulnerable to adverse effects of trade liberalisation than wealthier ones. We need better global governance concerning health and trade that better acknowledges and tackles the wide-ranging effects of trade on health. Indeed, we need better global governance in a variety of domains especially once we appreciate direct and indirect effects on human well-being. One such area is tax and accounting practices.

Third, reforming our international tax arrangements could be especially important in ensuring that everyone has the prospects for a decent life, which importantly includes enjoying access to decent healthcare. For every dollar of aid that goes to assist a developing country, approximately US$6–7 of corporate tax evasion flows out (Baker 2005). Many widespread currently legal practices facilitate massive tax escape, such as the use of tax havens, transfer pricing schemes (that allow goods to be traded at arbitrary prices in efforts to suggest large, untaxable losses are being incurred) or practices of non-disclosure of sales prices for resources (that greatly assist corrupt leaders in diverting revenue from developing countries for their own private use) (Brock 2009b: Chapter 5). Ensuring adequate revenue collection and tax compliance is important for development and democracy, in addition to ensuring developing countries can adequately fund essential goods such as healthcare. There are also several proposals concerning the imposition of global taxes that would improve health globally and have a reasonable chance of success and, in some cases, have already been implemented. The 'Air-Ticket Tax', operated by UNITAID, collects revenue that is used to address global health problems such as malaria, tuberculosis and AIDs (Brock 2009b: Chapter 5; Brock 2008: 161–84).

4. IDEAL WORLD JUSTICE, TRANSITIONAL JUSTICE AND REMEDIAL RESPONSIBILITIES: SOME FURTHER ANALYSIS

Given this brief survey of some practices and aspects of our international institutional arrangements, we see that there are many ways in which our current world order exacerbates poor global health. On many accounts of which are our strongest responsibilities, the most robust ones are so-called negative responsibilities, aimed at the prevention of harm. We all have negative duties to refrain from harming and therefore would seem to be squarely implicated in these health-harming practices when we participate in or uphold them, without taking steps to reform their most egregious aspects, especially when reasonable alternatives are available.

As the survey also highlights, there is an intimate connection between global health challenges and matters of social justice, which means we cannot isolate our responsibilities with respect to health in a way that does not deeply connect with many of our other justice responsibilities. As my analysis bears out, we cannot separate the responsibilities specific to health from the more general justice obligations we have, given the intimate connections between poor health and injustice. In an extended treatment elsewhere, I argue that global justice requires that all are adequately positioned to enjoy prospects for a decent life, which requires that we attend especially to enabling need satisfaction, protecting basic freedom, ensuring fair terms of cooperation in collective endeavours, and social and political arrangements that can underwrite these important goods are in place (Brock 2009b). All four of these components constitute the basis for grounding claims of entitlement and all four have important implications for health, just some of which are brought out in the analysis below.

As we see, many theorists draw attention to the ways in which we contribute to policies and activities that have significant health-harming effects. If, as Pogge, and Buchanan and DeCamp have argued, we have responsibilities not to contribute to activities that have significant health-harming effects, it seems we have a great many responsibilities. Will we indeed have too many? To give two examples: since weapons-trading or trade in cigarettes have health-harming effects, are we not culpable when we fail to change such trade practices? Are we morally culpable when we participate in a global economic order that upholds such practices? Perhaps we are indeed so culpable? Can we delimit a more manageable set of actions for which we are clearly more responsible? Should we try, or should we rather embrace the fact that our set of responsibilities here is large?

Let us begin the analysis by clarifying some issues. There are many agents who could potentially have responsibilities to move toward more just arrangements in our actual world. Many agents are involved in deciding, implementing and affecting policies that have health-harming effects. Examples of these different agents include governments, multinational corporations, consumers, investors or citizens. There might well be different kinds of responsibilities at the state, organisational and individual levels which track different kinds of activities or the nature of institutional involvement. Here I focus only on state-level responsibilities: the responsibilities citizens of one state owe to citizens of others, and describe some kinds of responsibilities they have with respect to health policy. I focus on governments and their responsibilities because governments are *de facto* the primary agents of justice in the world we currently inhabit. They are charged with the responsibilities to provide for and protect their citizens. Moreover, governments often act as efficient co-ordinators and dischargers of the responsibilities we have to one another as moral agents (Goodin 1998: 73–94). They are in an excellent position to co-ordinate and deliver on the responsibilities we all have to one another as human beings.

There are many levels at which we can engage with this question of responsibilities for health. We might be asking: in an ideal world, what responsibilities might we have with respect to health? Or, we could instead be asking a question such as this: in this non-ideal world, what responsibilities might we have with respect to health? Here I consider the question of transitional justice: how do we allocate responsibilities *in this world* for moving towards a more just one? So in this case: how should we allocate responsibilities for moving toward instantiating improvements in practices, policies and institutions that make progress toward our goals of improving global health? Who is responsible for making changes? Who, in short (and as I go on to explain), is responsible for showing moral leadership in initiating change? Here I argue that a large share of responsibility falls on the global advantaged to make necessary reforms (Pogge 2010: 187–9).[2] Typically that means that governments of affluent developed countries have some key responsibilities.

There are many kinds of responsibilities that could be in play when we talk about responsibilities with respect to poor health. David Miller draws a useful distinction between 'outcome' and 'remedial' responsibilities. Outcome responsibility is 'the responsibility we bear for our own actions and decisions' (Miller 2007: 81). By contrast, remedial responsibility is 'the responsibility we may have to come to the aid of those who need help' (Miller 2007: 81). Sometimes outcome and remedial responsibilities correspond, as when those who are responsible for poor decisions that result in harmful actions should go to the assistance of those adversely affected. But these do not always correspond well, for instance when the agents who are outcome responsible are no longer around, or are not in a position to help because, for instance, they are too poorly endowed to assist.

Both outcome and remedial responsibility have a role to play and are important in identifying and assigning responsibility. But they take quite different approaches: outcome responsibility 'starts with agents and asks how far they can reasonably be credited and debited with the results of their conduct' whereas, 'remedial responsibility starts with patients – people who are deprived or suffering – and asks who should shoulder the burden of helping them' (Miller 2007: 108).

According to Miller, 'an agent is outcome responsible for those consequences of his action that a reasonable person would have foreseen, given the circumstances' (Miller 2007: 96). He also offers us a useful connection theory of remedial responsibility. On this account, an agent, A, should be considered remedially responsible for the condition of a patient, P, when A is linked to P 'in one or more of the ways' specified below. There are six ways in which remedial responsibility can be identified:

Moral responsibility: On this dimension of responsibility, if A is morally responsible for P's condition, 'A must have acted in a way that displays moral fault: he must have deprived P deliberately or recklessly, or he must have failed to provide for P despite having a pre-existing obligation to do so (for example, he had promised to feed P, but then defaulted on his promise by doing nothing)' (Miller 2007: 100).

Outcome responsibility: A can be outcome responsible for P's plight without being morally responsible for it: perhaps P's situation is a consequence of an action that is completely morally neutral or even laudable. I open a better coffee shop than yours in the same neighbourhood with the result that your business fails. I am permitted to act in this way – it is morally neutral, *ceteris paribus*. But I am also outcome responsible for your predicament.

Causal responsibility: one can be causally responsible without being outcome responsible: I move backwards in a crowded train to avoid being crushed by someone moving forward and as a result knock over someone's package. I am causally but not necessarily outcome responsible here.

Benefit: A might have had no role in a process leading to P's deprivation (for instance, the first three ways discussed above), but might nonetheless have benefited from it. Benefiting from such a process might be sufficient to make A remedially responsible for helping P.

Capacity: Here the focus is on who is capable of assisting. There are actually two issues here: the effectiveness with which one can render aid and, second, the costs to the rectifier of remedying the situation. For instance, the strongest swimmer might be expected to effect the rescue, but only if this is also going to involve low cost to him. According to Miller, if 'A is uniquely in this position, then he is remedially responsible for P' (Miller 2007: 103).

Community: Consider the case of a child going missing. If she is from my village, or if there is some other relevant connection to her, I have more responsibility to look for her than others do.

On Miller's view, we certainly may hold contemporary citizens of democracies remedially responsible for actions performed on their behalf, including actions that have implications for non-citizens. So, what should we do about the case of assigning remedial responsibility for making changes to the global order? There are actually at least two issues here: there is the issue of responsibility for addressing harm already caused which determines who should directly assist those who currently suffer. But even more importantly, I believe, is the issue of who has responsibility for reforming the practices, institutions (and so forth) that perpetuate the situation that enables deprivation to continue. This is the question that primarily concerns me here. And it concerns me because most people in developed countries do not believe that they have responsibilities here to make changes, to take the initiative in reforms, or to show moral leadership. On the contrary, they typically act as if these matters are not their concern at all.

Let me discuss first why I think this is an issue of responsibility for moral leadership and the nature of the deep problems we face. This problem infects much international policy and it has the following structure:

(1) We have permissible international policies of a certain kind that have defects, especially in facilitating large-scale and important injustice.

(2) If we refrain from behaviours permitted by the policy on normative grounds, we put ourselves at a competitive disadvantage, since our competitors are not obliged to do so.

(3) It is, therefore, neither rational nor fair to expect us to so refrain.

(4) We would refrain from undesirable behaviours if we were obliged to do so or if we had an assurance that others would similarly refrain.

(5) So we would comply with a policy that required refraining from the undesirable practice.

(6) However, in the absence of a policy change, we have no substantial normative duties.

My claim is that this conclusion, (6), does not follow and, with the aid of an account of remedial responsibilities, we can show that, on the contrary, we have significant responsibilities to change the offending policy (or network of policies), under certain conditions.

States have responsibilities not to collude with or be accomplices in injustice. They could stop recognising the legitimacy of unjust regimes through engaging with them in 'business as usual', in continuing practices of trade, resource sales and the like. But many things states could and should do would place them in a disadvantageous position with respect to their competitors who may not be similarly inclined. Here I do not want to argue that states must always take the high road in our non-ideal world and sacrifice their interests for the sake of some conception of justice, *when no one else is doing anything remotely similar.* Rather, I argue for a different claim. In our non-ideal world, governments of affluent, developed states have at least some other responsibilities, I contend, namely, to show some moral leadership in mobilising for a more just network of international practices, rules and institutions. This will undoubtedly require time that could be spent on other goals, some disbursement of political capital, some expenditure of resources and soft power, not to mention opportunity costs and the like. But, I argue, this can be required in virtue of our remedial responsibilities, at least in certain cases. The view, then, is this:

> *Responsibilities to initiate change*: When an evidence-based case has been made that international practices, institutions, policies or agreements facilitate injustice, when reasonable modifications to these practices would not, governments of developed countries have special responsibilities to mobilise for changes to policies that would not contribute to injustice, under certain conditions such as when three key remedial connection factors apply (to be explained below).

We all have responsibilities not to participate in injustice. And in our non-ideal world, we, the global advantaged and especially our agents – governments – have special remedial responsibilities to show moral leadership in reforming such practices in virtue of several of the factors Miller identifies. Let us review. I pick out, more or less in descending order, the relevant factors by which this judgement is reached. As Miller notes, in some cases, benefiting from a process might be sufficient for agents to be held responsible for helping the deprived, even when there are no other salient connections between them. The dense network of arrangements characteristic of globalisation, some of which are surveyed above (such as concerning domains including trade, tax, accounting, recruitment, intellectual property rights or borrowing privileges), have benefited the global advantaged (the top 5 per cent of earners globally), which includes typical citizens of affluent, developed states (Pogge 2010: 187–9). In virtue of being in the top 5 per cent they are, by definition, better off than others to affect changes in virtue of disposable resources, leisure time and other resources necessary to make effective changes and to bear some costs (relative to our holdings). So both aspects of the capacity condition apply to them. Patterns of benefit coupled with capacity to make reforms might well be sufficient to make the case as to why they have important remedial responsibilities in these kinds of cases. But the case is strengthened further when we consider other criteria. The criterion of causal responsibility would also typically be satisfied on the view I defend. On my view, certain practices readily facilitate injustice. It is in this respect that the causal responsibility condition is met. Just as when I move backwards in a crowded train to avoid being crushed and knock someone's parcel over I may still be causally implicated, in the same way certain international practices facilitate important injustice, whether or not the moving train, the person coming towards me who forces me to step back (and so forth) might also be implicated. The moral responsibility criterion can also be invoked to strengthen the case, though here I will not put much weight on it so as not to have to defend this part of the argument (which is undertaken elsewhere) (Brock 2009b). I similarly will not appeal to any of the other criteria Miller discusses, though further analysis of these might yield additional support.

So, let us recap. At least in virtue of patterns of benefit, both ways in which we have strong capacity, and the way in which we facilitate injustice (the causal dimension), we have sufficient grounds for assigning remedial responsibility to citizens of affluent, developed states, and particularly their governments, who act as agents on their behalf, to take a leading role in initiating the relevant changes. *Ceteris paribus*, those states that have derived more benefits and have greater capacities to remedy defects are more obligated to show moral leadership in making necessary reforms, especially when their actions have also facilitated more injustice.

Here I leave to one side some tricky issues, such as what kinds of evidence-based cases meet the threshold of acceptability. I believe the threshold is met in many of the examples highlighted in sections 2 and 3 above, such as showing how our current arrangements in several domains are defective (including practices surveyed earlier concerning taxation arrangements, accounting and disclosure requirements – or lack thereof, borrowing and resource privileges, intellectual property rights, and recruitment practices, especially as reasonable reforms to such practices are all available, as is documented in some detail) (Pogge 2008c; Brock 2009b). The central point of this argument is anyhow a conceptual one: I aim to rebut a particular source of apathy, namely the view that developed countries have no responsibilities to reform institutions. I argue, on the contrary, that they have special responsibilities to do just that in virtue of their remedial responsibilities.

In determining our more specific responsibilities, we are bound to confront difficult cases, such as whether our obligations extend to reforming all practices that facilitate injustice, such as to prohibit trade in weapons or perhaps even trade in cigarettes. Arguably, some trade in weapons is beneficial when it allows governments to protect their citizens better. Though defences on behalf of trade in cigarettes seem notably absent, perhaps however, like many other goods, consumption of cigarettes in small quantities or even moderation does not necessarily undermine health, and if (for instance) the social practice of smoking with others enhances community-building, indirect health benefits may accrue to some. I will not take a stand on those issues here as I believe there are more detrimental and worrisome practices that require more urgent reform and facilitate more pervasive, large-scale injustice. I submit, there are many clear cases where our failure to act is more clearly worrying. So we fail in our remedial responsibilities when we fail to reform taxation practices that perpetuate tax escape that undermine governments' abilities to provide adequate healthcare, public goods and other essentials requisite to a minimally decent functioning society. And we fail in these responsibilities when we do not make necessary changes to healthcare recruitment that strips countries of their healthcare personnel, leaving them woefully understaffed. And we fail miserably when we continue to implement trade liberalisation policies that undermine food security or allow massive levels of starvation and malnutrition to result. And the insistence on repayment of debts undertaken by repressive regimes no longer in power, which strips public coffers of funds to devote to healthcare, education, infrastructure, transportation and the like, is yet a further failure of our remedial responsibilities, as is our failure to reform the TRIPS agreements which perpetuate massive under-funding for diseases that affect the great majority of people. In such cases we will have our work cut out for us, and showing moral leadership in initiating and co-operating with others similarly placed to introduce reforms will keep us busy enough for the time being.

Notes

1. Similarly, although anthropogenic climate change will affect all human beings, it will affect the poorest and most disadvantaged much more greatly. Some of the pathways that will lead to health inequities include the fact that extreme weather events are likely to increase, resulting in more general destruction, flooding, infectious disease or food shortages, all of which affect those with fewer resources more greatly than the better-resourced. Sea level rises, drought, water insecurity and human relocation are other mechanisms through which it can be predicted that the more vulnerable will suffer disproportionate effects.
2. The global advantaged would include the top 5 per cent of global income earners. They have enjoyed plentiful benefits during the period of globalisation that currently characterises our world. For some evidence that they have enjoyed remarkable benefits, see, for instance, Pogge (2010: 187–9). The top 5 per cent have greatly increased their considerable advantage even more strikingly over the last twenty years than in previous ones.

Chapter 7

OUTLINING THE GLOBAL DUTIES OF JUSTICE OWED TO WOMEN LIVING WITH HIV/AIDS IN SUB-SAHARAN AFRICA

Angela Kaida and Patti Tamara Lenard

Maternal mortality is the world's worst health inequity. Every day a thousand women die from preventable causes related to pregnancy and childbirth; 99 per cent of these maternal deaths occur in developing countries (World Health Organization 2010). There is a 400-fold difference in the Maternal Mortality Ratio (MMR) between the country with the highest MMR (Afghanistan MMR = 1,575 maternal deaths per 100,000 live births) and the country with the lowest MMR (Italy MMR = 4 maternal deaths per 100,000 live births). Recent reviews of progress on improving maternal health reveal a positive trend toward fewer global maternal deaths, from 526,000 in 1980 to 342,900 in 2008 (Hogan et al. 2010). This decrease was observed across all countries and regions with one notable exception, sub-Saharan Africa, where the MMR *increased* over time and accounts for over half (52 per cent) of global maternal deaths. The primary reason driving this trend is the large, feminised HIV epidemics in the region. Without HIV (or, arguably, with universal access to antiretroviral treatment services), annual maternal deaths would have been 20 per cent lower in 2008 (that is, 61,000 excess maternal deaths per year due to HIV). The starkness of this finding led the editor of *The Lancet* to conclude that 'the connection between HIV and maternal health is now explicitly laid bare' (Horton 2010).

In this chapter we argue perhaps unsurprisingly that cosmopolitan principles, as applied to this case, show why it is that wealthy nations bear responsibility for remedying the conditions under which this epidemic is permitted to persist. We begin with an account of the HIV/AIDS epidemic in sub-Saharan Africa and we justify our particular focus on the struggles women face in this region. We then spend the bulk of the chapter refuting the three main reasons given to justify ignoring this specific health inequity: 1) wealthy nations do not have the resources with which to make a difference; 2) wealthy nations are not responsible for the havoc wreaked by the disease; and 3) the mechanism by which HIV is transmitted is well known, and therefore those who contract the disease are by and large victims of bad choices (rather than bad luck), and therefore the responsibility that wealthy nations might have to remedy gross health inequities is mitigated in this case. All three of these reasons are intended to deny the responsibility that wealthy nations have to remedy the HIV/AIDS epidemic in sub-Saharan Africa; our general project is to show that in fact responsibility does fall to those who are able to offer aid in this case. We shall, over the course of this discussion, consider how responsibility should be assigned under non-ideal conditions.

To begin, it is worth noting the very simple cosmopolitan principles on which we rely; these have been detailed in earlier chapters in general, and as they apply to health in particular (see Garrett Wallace Brown's and Gillian Brock's chapters in particular): 1) all people are of equal moral worth; 2) as a result of which we owe duties of justice to others; and 3) no one should be faced with undue disadvantage as a result of factors that are arbitrary from a moral point of view, including, for example, religion, race, culture and, in our cases in particular, gender and nationality (Tan 2004; Caney 2005; Brock 2009b).

OVERVIEW OF THE GLOBAL HIV/AIDS PANDEMIC

In 2010, at the cusp of the fourth decade of the HIV pandemic, the global community welcomed new statistics suggesting a 'turning of the tide' in its course: fewer people are becoming infected with HIV and fewer people are dying from the disease (UNAIDS 2010). Now, more than ever, we are being challenged to envision and create a new future for HIV: 'Zero new HIV infections. Zero discrimination. Zero AIDS-related deaths'(UNAIDS 2010). This renewed optimism is tempered by the fact that HIV remains the most difficult and globally devastating infectious agent of our history and each year more people are newly infected than are being initiated onto life-saving antiretroviral treatment. Sustaining and advancing the hard-fought, fragile successes against the spread and impact of HIV/AIDS demands focused, evidence-based, appropriately resourced and results-oriented action.

Preventing and mitigating the impact of HIV/AIDS constitutes a critical strategy toward improving global development and building a more prosperous and equitable global society. In September 2000, world leaders at the United Nations adopted eight Millennium Development Goals (MDGs), which articulated measurable development goals to be reached by 2015 (United Nations 2000). The global development relevance of HIV/AIDS was captured in its dedicated MDG (targets 6a and 6b), which assigned concrete, measurable goals to halt and to begin to reverse the spread of HIV/AIDS and to achieve universal access to antiretroviral treatment (ART) for HIV/AIDS for all those in need (UNAIDS 2010). As we inch toward the 2015 deadline for achieving the MDGs, however, the global HIV community is witnessing stagnating levels of global resourcing and waning political leadership for continuing the fight against HIV. Rather than focusing on means to support and leverage the fragile, recent and unprecedented successes of the global HIV/AIDS response, misguided calls have denounced 'AIDS exceptionalism' and are urging diversion of resources and attention from HIV/AIDS to other global health concerns (Ahmed et al. 2009).

This concerning trend has underscored the need to rearticulate the scientific and moral grounds for sustained global leadership and financial commitment to addressing HIV/AIDS as a global public health priority. Such a strategy must continue to emphasise the scale and impact of the pandemic and recapitulate the remarkable scientific and social innovation developed to reduce the global incidence and consequence of HIV infection. Importantly, the response must also speak clearly to the obligations that wealthy countries have to address the profound global inequities determining and exacerbating HIV/AIDS in developing countries.

A FOCUS ON WOMEN

With women accounting for over half of the world's 33.3 million people living with HIV and an increasing proportion of incident infections each year, there is clear evidence of the feminisation of poverty in general, and of the global HIV pandemic in particular (Jaggar 2002; UNAIDS 2010). The vast majority live in sub-Saharan Africa, where over 12 million women are currently living with HIV, accounting for 61 per cent of the region's HIV-infected adult population. The gender disparity in the distribution of HIV is even more pronounced among

SUB-SAHARAN AFRICA		Adults and children living with HIV	Adults and children newly infected with HIV	% Adult prevalence (15–49 years)	AIDS-related deaths among adults and children
	2009	22.5 million [20.9–24.2 million]	1.8 million [1.6–2.0 million]	5.0 [4.7–5.2]	1.3 million [1.1–1.5 million]
	2001	20.3 million [18.9–21.7 million]	2.2 million [1.9–2.4 million]	5.9 [5.6–6.1]	1.4 million [1.2–1.6 million]

Figure 7.1 Number of adults and children newly infected and living with HIV, and number of AIDS-related deaths in sub-Saharan Africa, 2001 and 2009 (UNAIDS 2010).

youth, as young women 15–24 years of age are up to eight times more likely than young men to be HIV-positive (UNAIDS 2010). HIV/AIDS remains the leading cause of mortality among women of reproductive age and is responsible for more than 50 per cent of mortality in five sub-Saharan African countries with the highest HIV prevalence.

The reasons for women's disproportionate burden of disease relate to their greater physiologic and social susceptibility to HIV acquisition (Quinn and Overbaugh 2005). Physiologically, women are at least twice as likely as men to become infected with HIV during unprotected sex, in large part because they are the receptive sexual partner and expose the large surface area of the vaginal mucosal membrane to infection during and after intercourse. HIV concentration is higher in semen than in vaginal fluid, further increasing the male-to-female risk of transmission. Physiologic vulnerability is exacerbated among younger women since the immature vaginal tract is more susceptible to abrasion during intercourse, increasing opportunity for HIV entry (Quinn and Overbaugh 2005).

Compounding the greater physiologic susceptibility is the unequal distribution of the socio-economic and structural determinants of health (for example, poverty, gender inequity, gender-based violence, low health literacy) and prevailing harmful cultural practices (for example, female genital cutting, child marriage, widow inheritance) that increase women's vulnerability to HIV infection and its consequences. Prevailing and systemic social, financial and power inequalities that increase women's dependence on men for financial and other support and limit women's control and negotiating power over condom use and other behavioural HIV prevention strategies, place women at increased risk of HIV infection (UNAIDS 2010). Acknowledging these broader reasons for women's disproportionate vulnerability to HIV is essential to inform why we should act and how we should act to address this health inequity.

The focus on women and HIV/AIDS is justified not only in virtue of their greater susceptibility to the disease. Additionally, there are complications of the disease faced uniquely by women in virtue of their role as child-bearers and therefore generating a focus not solely on women's health but on women's *reproductive* health. Globally, the primary mode of transmission of HIV is unprotected heterosexual intercourse, which entangles and exacerbates the relationship between the epidemic and women's reproductive health. HIV infection among women of reproductive age raises individual clinical care and public health concerns about the incidence of pregnancy. The first of these concerns relates to the health and survival of the mother. In the absence of effective treatment, HIV-positive women have lower life expectancy and higher morbidity than HIV-negative women (Nunn et al. 1997). The risk of maternal mortality is exacerbated among HIV-positive women, with reports indicating that HIV-related maternal deaths have increased dramatically in regions with high HIV prevalence among women of reproductive age (National Committee on Confidential Enquiries into Maternal Deaths 2003).

The second concern relates to the risks of HIV transmission to sero-discordant sexual partners for the purposes of conception or otherwise (where one partner is HIV positive and the other is HIV negative). The vast majority of conceptions occur without the use of reproductive technologies such as sperm-washing and artificial insemination. Thus, the unprotected sexual activity required for conception carries a risk of HIV transmission to uninfected sexual partners.

Third, reproduction among HIV-positive women also carries a risk of vertical transmission during pregnancy, labour and through breast-feeding, commonly known as Mother-to-Child Transmission (MTCT). Without optimal therapy and intervention, the risk of transmitting HIV from a mother to a baby ranges from 12 to 45 per cent, depending on the setting and individual circumstances. With optimal treatment and intervention, however, the risk of MTCT drops to less than 2 per cent, as seen in North American and European settings (Cooper et al. 2002).

Adequately addressing the reproductive needs of women living with HIV is a critical strategy towards mitigating the impact of the HIV epidemic as well as reducing maternal and infant mortality. However, the prevailing under-emphasis of HIV within reproductive health programming (and vice versa) is evident in the numbers. Each year the absolute number of pregnancies among women living with HIV in sub-Saharan Africa exceeds 1.4 million (World Health Organization 2009), of which an estimated 50–84 per cent are unintended (Desgrees-Du-Lou et al. 2002; Rochat et al. 2006; Laher et al. 2009). Many of these pregnancies contribute to distressing adverse outcomes for women, children and their families. Every year nearly 350,000 infants are infected with HIV via vertical transmission (UNAIDS 2010). In addition, across sub-Saharan Africa there are an estimated 8.9 million maternal orphans due to HIV/AIDS-associated mortality (UNAIDS 2004). Moreover, there are an estimated 2 million new adult HIV infections each year, overwhelmingly related to unprotected sexual intercourse.

While the global health community has expressed the financial willingness and provided international statements of the commitment to make a difference on maternal and child health, it must be made clear that achieving this goal is linked to the fight against HIV. The increasingly popular trend of lobbying to divert funding and resourcing away from HIV/AIDS will severely undermine any well-intentioned global maternal and child health strategy. Such a strategy may also lead to treatment interruption and refusal for people living with HIV yielding a potential re-increase in entirely avoidable, premature deaths, as well as higher rates of vertical and sexual transmission of HIV. From an evidence-based, scientific and, crucially, moral perspective, diverting funds from HIV prevention and treatment efforts, especially among women in sub-Saharan Africa, is unjustifiable.

REFUTING OBJECTIONS

There is considerable reluctance to accept the claims, which find their foundation in cosmopolitan principles, that the vast inequalities that separate the wealthiest nations from the poorest nations are a matter of justice that imposes duties on the wealthiest of nations. As many of the chapters have noted, the duties imposed specifically by health inequalities are difficult to articulate and often do not find more general widespread acceptance. Instead, the tendency is to ascribe responsibility for health outcomes either to the individuals affected or to the domestic environment in which these individuals find themselves. We do not have space to consider these debates in more depth here, however, and instead our objective is to show that three common and powerful ways in which wealthy nations deny responsibility for women living with HIV/AIDS are not persuasive, thus leading us to conclude that they possess duties of justice in the case at issue in this chapter.

Objection 1: The resources available are inadequate

It is common to claim that resource scarcity prevents wealthy nations from contributing more aggressively to remedying inequalities in general and health inequalities in particular.[1] Resource scarcity comes in at least two forms: financial and scientific. That is, in claiming resource scarcity as a reason to avoid contributing more to remedying health inequalities, wealthy nations may be claiming one or both of inadequate material resources or inadequate scientific/technological resources. A variation on this claim is that other dimensions of inequalities are themselves more pressing, or that health inequalities are simply a manifestation of other inequalities. These claims serve ultimately to justify the refusal to take responsibility for what are plainly appalling inequalities. Yet, as we'll argue, advances in providing treatment for people living with HIV belie the claim that inadequate resources, material or scientific/technological, are to blame for the ongoingness of the epidemic. We have effective and cost-effective scientific, social and pharmacological resources to combat the progression and ongoing transmission of HIV (Creese et al. 2002; Johnston et al. 2010; Johri and Ako-Arrey 2011).

By suppressing HIV viral load, appropriate and sustained use of antiretroviral therapy (ART), the standard treatment regimen for HIV infection, significantly increases life expectancy and decreases morbidity among HIV-infected individuals (Hogg et al. 1997; Frank J. Palella Jr. et al. 1998; Hogg et al. 1998; Hogg et al. 2001). Worldwide and across all countries, AIDS deaths have begun to decline (UNAIDS 2010). The effects of antiretroviral therapy are highly evident in sub-Saharan Africa, where an estimated 320,000 (or 20 per cent) fewer people died of AIDS-related causes in 2009 than in 2004 (UNAIDS 2010).

In addition to the clinical and survival benefits, expanding access to ART dramatically reduces the risk of mother-to-child transmission to less than 2 per cent (Cooper et al. 2002). Countries across eastern and southern Africa have reported declines in incidence of vertical transmission and infant and under-five mortality after the introduction of Prevention of Mother-to-Child transmission (PMTCT) services (World Health Organization 2009). Provision of ART also reduces risk of HIV transmission to discordant sexual partners, which thereby supports HIV prevention efforts (Montaner et al. 2006). Under the 'Treatment as Prevention' premise, achieving the commitment to universal access to HIV treatment will have a multiplicative effect since it will save individual lives of people living with HIV and will significantly reduce the risk of transmission. The cost-effectiveness of this strategy has recently been demonstrated (Johnston et al. 2010).

There is also clear evidence that scaling-up access to HIV prevention, care and treatment services and the associated investments in health infrastructure have had additional positive impacts on human resources for health, improved laboratory monitoring and pharmacy capacity, and more effective health management information systems (Embrey et al. 2009; Justman et al. 2009). Moreover, the scale-up of HIV-related services has positively impacted numerous other women and child health outcomes, including increases in antenatal care use, attendance at clinics and hospitals for deliveries, vaccinations, increased contraceptive use, treatment of sexually transmitted infections and diagnosis of tuberculosis (Walton et al. 2005).

The provision of global resources to fight HIV began in earnest in 2001, with the creation of the Global Fund to Fight AIDS, Tuberculosis and Malaria (Global Fund), which was followed by the US President's Emergency Plan for AIDS Relief (PEPFAR) in 2003. In light of these funding announcements, at the G8 summit in Gleneagles, Scotland in 2005, the global community made an unprecedented commitment to achieving universal access to HIV treatment and care to people around the world by 2010.

In the years between 2002 and 2009, we witnessed an unprecedented global effort directed at increasing access to ART for people living with HIV in sub-Saharan Africa and other resource-limited settings. The scale-up process has been dramatic; by the end of 2009, 5,254,000 people were receiving antiretroviral therapy in low- and middle-income countries, an increase of over 1.2 million people from December 2008. This represents a 30 per cent rise from a year earlier and a 13-fold increase in six years (World Health Organization 2010).

Most of the increase occurred in sub-Saharan Africa where, in 2009, nearly four million HIV-infected people were receiving HAART, accounting for an estimated 37 per cent of those in need of treatment. The region accounts for 72 per cent of the estimated treatment need in low- and middle-income countries, and 74 per cent of the total number of people receiving treatment. In addition, some 54 per cent of pregnant women living with HIV in the region received ART to prevent HIV transmission to their infants, of whom nearly 10 per cent were receiving HAART for their own health (World Health Organization 2010). While there remains a high level of unmet need, this level of antiretroviral coverage represents a substantial increase from previous years. Between 2007 and 2008 alone, nearly one million more HIV-infected individuals in need of treatment in sub-Saharan Africa commenced antiretroviral therapy.

The scale-up of access to HIV treatment and care is the result of remarkable scientific and social innovation coupled with global advocacy and political commitment to implementing strategies that we know make a difference to preventing and mitigating the consequences of HIV infection. Numerous countries are actively demonstrating that achieving the G8's stated goals of universal access to HIV treatment and care is possible (World Health Organization 2010).

In other words, we have good reason to be sceptical of the 'resource scarcity' claim as an explanation for the failure of wealthy nations to take responsibility for providing aid to women living with HIV/AIDS in sub-Saharan Africa. Overall, we have ample evidence of the scientific and technological resource capacity to achieve universal access to HIV prevention, care and treatment and to address the risks and consequences of HIV infection.

Objection 2: Those who are in a position to help are not responsible for the crisis

It is commonly claimed that one bears responsibility for remedying a wrong only when one has caused that wrong. If I steal from someone, it is my responsibility to return what I've stolen; if I slap someone, it is my responsibility to remedy the harm I've caused. Yet, in the case at issue – maternal mortality as a result of HIV/AIDS – a standard response is that 'we' have not caused the epidemic, and although it is egregious, and while we may choose to extend aid to communities that are struggling with the consequences of it, we are not responsible as a matter of justice to devote our resources to alleviating it. We are only responsible for remedying harm on this view, if we are causally responsible for having produced it in the first place. Yet, there are three reasons to deny the plausibility of this objection.

First, as Gillian Brock outlined in an earlier chapter, those who are in the position to offer aid may have the duty to offer this aid. Citing David Miller's categorisation of the varieties of responsibility, she observes that we may have duties of remedial responsibility – that is, of justice – to offer aid where we can do so, simply in virtue of our capacity to do so (Miller 2007). If our argument above is persuasive, then, and our scepticism of the 'resource scarcity' claim is reasonable, wealthy nations have remedial responsibilities to offer aid in the case at issue here.

Second, the denial of responsibility for health inequalities that face 'them' over 'there' relies on an at least partially inaccurate understanding of how moral responsibilities are allocated in a global world that is characterised by sovereign nation-states. For some anti-cosmopolitan scholars, the boundaries that divide states divide humanity into associations that more or less are responsible for themselves and themselves alone (Miller 2005; Nagel 2005). On this view, that one state (or several states) suffers from a health epidemic is of no (moral) concern to another; duties of justice apply only within associations, and state boundaries serve to identify the associations in which these duties apply. This view is unfortunately prevalent among many.

Yet, led by theorising by cosmopolitan thinkers, many others have argued that, while it is true that duties of justice apply only within the boundaries of associations – a view sometimes termed 'associationalism' – the increasing interdependence that characterises the global community is such that denying that nations are increasingly interconnected and interdependent is disingenuous. Instead, many argue, we should understand that as interconnections and interdependence increase among nations, the duties we have to those with whom we share these new, global associations likewise increase. In particular, as these interconnections increase, and therefore as the global association expands and deepens, it becomes increasingly difficult to justify inequalities – in our case, health inequalities – among those who are now, in effect, members of a shared association (Caney 2011).

Both reasons identified above, however, assume that no action has been taken by those who are in the position to offer help and explain why they are morally obligated to do so, even though they are not implicated in causing the wrong. And while we agree that wealthy nations have duties simply because they are in the position to aid, and while we agree that the global association is sufficiently deep to justify the claim that duties of justice are owed throughout the association, in fact we also believe that wealthy nations have taken responsibility-inducing actions that require them to focus on aiding women living with HIV/AIDS. In particular, as we have outlined, their acknowledgement through a variety of international organisations of the depth of the crisis in sub-Saharan Africa, especially as it applies to women, and their attendant stated commitments to which they have not yet lived up, are such that they generate responsibilities; the act of promising to offer aid generates the duty to do so (Scheffler 2003b). Nations in sub-Saharan Africa have raised their expectations of aid as a result of a series of public pronouncements by wealthy nations, outlining their commitments to those who are suffering. Wealthy nations have in other words already intervened in ways that suggest that they understand that they are responsible to aid; more importantly, their public pronouncements and their stated commitments are such that they have produced, in sub-Saharan African nations, an expectation of aid, and actions that are consistent with such an expectation.

In particular, despite tremendous progress, we are less than half way towards achieving the goal of universal access to HIV treatment and care to people around the world and have already passed the 2010 deadline set by G8 leaders at the Gleneagles meeting. During the recent Global Fund replenishment meeting, donors committed US$11.7 billion for the years 2011–13 to achieving the MDGs related to HIV, malaria and tuberculosis. This amount, while substantial, falls far short of what was originally promised. Indeed, the pledged amount remains approximately one-third of the UNAIDS estimate of the resources actually needed to achieve universal access. The initial pledge (and repeated promises) by G8 leaders to achieve universal access was based on solid scientific evidence and was a response to the growing demands for global action on HIV. Countries and individuals who rely on the promised assistance for addressing HIV in their regions could reasonably have expected these commitments to have been made in good faith and global leaders can be expected to honour commitments already made.

In 2010, the year that the pledge to universal access ought to have been realised, the G8 held another summit in Muskoka, Canada. At this summit, the Canadian government announced that the G8's signature initiative under the Canadian presidency would be to address the desperate state of maternal and child health in developing countries. As part of this new initiative, G8 member nations committed to spend collectively an additional $5 billion between 2010 and 2015 to accelerate progress toward the achievement of Millennium Development Goals 4 and 5, the reduction of maternal death, infant mortality and child mortality in developing countries. Shortly after the Muskoka meeting, in September 2010, world leaders gathered at the UN Millennium Development Goal summit to review progress made on achieving the MDGs and announced financial commitments of $40 billion toward achieving the goals, with again a particular emphasis on reducing maternal and child deaths.

Addressing the critical state of maternal and child health around the world is a pre-requisite for achieving the remaining MDGs. These global public health priorities were in desperate need of additional resources and focused attention to achieve the stated goals, and our global leadership should be lauded for their commitment to these causes. Largely under-emphasised in these announcements, however, is that HIV/AIDS remains the leading cause of death for women of child-bearing age globally and remains a critical barrier to achieving progress on maternal and child health. Moreover, that previous commitments to universal access to HIV prevention, care and treatment should have been fulfilled as an essential component to addressing maternal and child health in developing countries, but have not been, is also underemphasised.

Thus, although wealthy nations may not be causally responsible for the HIV/AIDS crisis, their actions – effectively, promises – are such that they have generated the duty to work toward remedying it.

Objection 3: Those who contract HIV/AIDS are guilty of bad choices

A final objection takes us into the details of the egalitarian thinking that underpins cosmopolitan political theory. This objection suggests that those who contract HIV/AIDS are guilty of bad choices, and that those who suffer as a result of the bad choices they've made are not entitled to aid. On this view, infected women are akin to the 'imprudent' that occupy so much luck egalitarian philosophising, since they may be expected to know that the actions they take can lead to their own infection (see Adina Preda's chapter for a discussion of the relevance of imprudence in identifying whether we have a right to health in the first place). For luck egalitarians, crudely described, one should not be responsible for situations in which one finds oneself as a matter of luck ('brute luck') but one should be responsible for the choices one makes ('option luck') (Dworkin 2000). To the extent that women can be viewed as 'making a choice', then, and acquire HIV, they are the victims of bad option luck. The outside community bears no duties of justice toward these women who are simply victims of bad option luck. As Preda describes in her chapter, this is often an uncomfortable result, since many communities do feel that they are responsible for coming to the aid of those who are the victims of bad option luck: offering medical care to smokers who contract lung cancer, or to helmet-less motorcycle victims, are two standard examples deployed to illustrate this intuition.

Our objective here is not to comment on the merits of what is a technical dispute among luck egalitarians, but rather to illustrate how this common distinction – between choice and luck – serves to highlight the difficulties of characterising the situation faced by women living with HIV/AIDS in sub-Saharan Africa. In doing so, we draw on recent discussions of whether responsibility-inducing choice can be attributed to those who make decisions in non-optimal conditions, which is surely an understatement when describing the conditions under which women in sub-Saharan Africa make decisions (for example, limited access to women-controlled HIV prevention options, socio-cultural environment that marginalises women and limits their ability to negotiate safer sexual practices, poverty and financial dependence, violations to human and sexual rights, and high risk of sexual and gender-based violence) that lead them to acquire HIV infection.

Following the standard choice–luck distinction, we have two ways in which to evaluate women's situation in sub-Saharan Africa. On one interpretation, as above, women are the victims of their own bad choices. They may know that sexual contact with those who are infected can result in HIV/AIDS (for the purposes of this argument, let us assume that they do have this information, which is certainly not true of most of the women concerned (Bunnell et al. 2006)), and they may know or suspect that their partners are likely to be infected (again, for the purposes of this argument, let us assume that they have this information, which is certainly not the norm for many women concerned). If this were the right way to characterise the conditions under which women are infected, we might well conclude that they are responsible for their infections, and therefore any aid we offer them is a matter of charity rather than justice.

On a second interpretation, the fact that women are born to communities in which HIV/AIDS is rampant, and therefore that the likelihood that they become infected with the disease is higher than it is elsewhere, is a matter of morally arbitrary luck. Earlier we outlined the critical and prevailing socio-economic and structural determinants that shape the lives of women in sub-Saharan Africa and thus make them more vulnerable to contracting HIV/AIDS, which range from extreme poverty to the prevalence of gender-based violence to low literacy to cultural practices that are harmful to women. Since we do not choose where we are born, the conditions into which we are born are not our 'fault' and therefore look more like 'bad brute luck'. On this view, the fact that women contract HIV/AIDS in known risky encounters – even though they may be aware of the risks associated with their actions – is not something for which they can be held responsible.

At first glance, each of these proposals is evidently problematic. In the first, it seems mistaken to attribute the contraction of HIV to choice in such a way that outsiders are not duty-bound to come to her aid. Doing so ignores the context in which marginalised women in sub-Saharan Africa must make decisions, that is, a context in which the options they have may be frighteningly small and sub-optimal. In the second, it seems we run the danger of denying the autonomy of women who make choices in difficult circumstances. By refusing to attribute responsibility to them for their actions – by 'blaming' the conditions in which they act on the structural conditions that shape their options – we run the risk of denying that these women are autonomous and rational decision-makers. Yet, the second solution is more promising: it promises in particular to make, as Zofia Stemplowska has argued, questions of justice sensitive to responsibility (Stemplowska 2009). On this interpretation, whether an individual can be said to be responsible for her actions – in the sense of being required to bear the costs of the disadvantage that she acquires as a result – depends in large part on the background conditions in which she acts. If, as seems clear, the background in which women in sub-Saharan Africa act is such that their options are severely constrained, that they knowingly engage in risky behaviour is not sufficient to deem them responsible for the consequences of their actions.

However, the objective is not to deny the autonomy of the women involved. Rather, the point is to acknowledge that, given the conditions in which these women are forced to make decisions, they cannot be taken to be responsible for their actions in such a way that the duties of justice that others possess to help them are avoided. We can see, for instance, the distinction between the case of women who contract HIV in sub-Saharan Africa, under conditions of highly constrained options, and the case of the mountain-climber who chooses against purchasing insurance in advance of a dangerous climb, and then finds himself stranded and in need of rescue. Only the mountain-climber is responsible for bearing the costs of the disadvantages he has incurred as a result of his decision. We are duty-bound, however, to offer aid to HIV-infected women in sub-Saharan Africa.

MOVING THE FOCUS TO ACCESS TO ANTIRETROVIRAL TREATMENT

We can see therefore that women in sub-Saharan Africa face two distinct injustices in need of remedy: one injustice arises simply in virtue of their having been born in environments that are less able, for a range of reasons, to protect them from acquiring HIV, and another arises in virtue of their inability to access the drugs they need in order to reduce the likelihood that they contract the disease, to slow its progression, and to prevent it being passed on to their children and to sero-negative sexual partners.

In our view, shifting to a focus on access to ART serves to focus the justice concerns where they belong – on those who are failing to carry out the duties they have toward others. It is a mistake to focus on the alleged responsibility that women may carry for having contracted the disease. Instead, as we have argued, the conditions under which the disease is contracted are such that they belie the claim that women are themselves responsible to suffer from the particular disadvantages they face as a result of contracting HIV/AIDS. The focus on treatment provision to HIV-infected women serves to identify the locus of the duties that are not being carried out adequately, that is, by those who have the ability to help and by those who have pledged to do so.

Our chapter began with an account of the struggles faced by women infected with HIV/AIDS in sub-Saharan Africa; there we observed that women's biological susceptibility to the disease and the socio-economic conditions under which they live conspire to make them particularly vulnerable to the contraction of HIV/AIDS. We then argued that two common objections, which are deployed to deny the responsibility that wealthy nations have to come to the aid of these women, are not persuasive. One objection simply denied that wealthy nations carry duties of justice in this case; from a moral point of view, these women are not members of the same association as they are, and since duties of justice only apply within associations, no duties of justice apply here. Another objection suggested that wealthy nations are mistakenly thought to have the resources necessary to carry out these duties. In both cases, we argued that these objections were implausible. In the first, we argued that the connections that increasingly bind nations have produced a global environment that can readily be described as an association, across which duties of justice apply. In the second, we argued that the very fact that wealthy nations have pledged to provide ART to those who need it and that recent history has suggested the ability to scale up the provision of ART efficiently, combine to deny the claim that resource scarcity now justifies ignoring or deprioritising the plight of women in sub-Saharan Africa. Finally, we considered the possibility that women who contract HIV/AIDS do so *knowingly* and are therefore justifiably required to bear the consequences of the disease; we denied, however, that there is plausibility to this claim. While women may have the information they need to understand that they are making risky decisions, we observed that the structural conditions that persist in sub-Saharan Africa are such that they are not often able to act in such a way as to prevent their contraction of the disease. These structural conditions are such that women in sub-Saharan Africa cannot justifiably be required to bear the consequences of having contracted HIV/AIDS. We concluded just above, by briefly noting the importance of focusing not on whether responsibility lies with the women who contract HIV/AIDS but instead on the responsibility that wealthy nations have to provide access to ART. In sum, we have attempted to show that cosmopolitan political principles – which emphasise the equal moral worth of all individuals, the duties of justice which we therefore owe to others, and the fact that the 'health conditions' in which we find ourselves is a matter of moral luck – report definitively that the duties to respond to the HIV/AIDS crisis that has befallen women in sub-Saharan Africa fall squarely on the shoulders of the most wealthy nations.

Note

1. The frequency with which we hear that the global community possesses inadequate resources to deal with the most pressing of inequalities was observed by Ted Schrecker, one of the contributors to the workshop which ultimately gave rise to this volume.

Part 3

Measuring Health and Health Outcomes

Chapter 8

MEASURING GLOBAL HEALTH[1]

Kristin Voigt

INTRODUCTION

Summary measures of population health combine information about morbidity and premature mortality within a single 'metric'. Particularly prominent at the international level is the Global Burden of Disease (GBD) study, which uses disability-adjusted life-years (DALYs) to quantify the disease burden resulting from different health conditions across the world. The study aims to provide an objective assessment of the state of global health, capturing not only premature mortality but also the burden of non-fatal health conditions. Moreover, the measure can – and was explicitly designed to – inform policy decisions relating to global health, particularly about priority-setting and resource allocation. For example, the Disease Control Priorities Project uses GBD data to make health policy recommendations for developing countries.

From the beginning of the project, the salience of normative questions in designing an appropriate measure of global health was apparent. These questions were addressed explicitly in the development of the GBD approach and were the focus of much of the criticism voiced against the GBD and its methodology. This chapter focuses on the influence that concerns about the effects of global health measures on health policy have had on the development of the GBD methodology. The GBD researchers emphasise that when health indicators gain prominence, they inevitably have an influence on policy debates and decisions. It is incumbent on those developing such indicators to recognise this 'normative shadow' and to design health measures in such a way that their influence on policy is unproblematic. In particular, we must anticipate how health measures could lead to unfair decisions with respect to resource allocation or priority-setting, and attempt to prevent such effects. This chapter outlines how such concerns have influenced different aspects of the GBD methodology. Designing health measures so that they reflect concerns about fairness may, however, create conceptual tensions and distort our understanding of the burden of disease; the chapter assesses the significance of this conceptual problem for the GBD project. Finally, I consider different strategies for enhancing the DALY's role as a tool in policy decisions and outline the direction implicit in recent revisions of the GBD methodology.

THE GLOBAL BURDEN OF DISEASE (GBD) PROJECT

The Global Burden of Disease project was initiated in the early 1990s. Two primary aims were pursued through this project. First, there was concern about the fact that health policy was informed primarily by information about mortality rates, particularly among children, and did not pay due attention to the effects of disability and non-fatal disease. The GBD project set out to combine information about both mortality and morbidity into a single measure to provide a fuller picture of the state of global health (Murray 1996). Thus, the GBD allows for comparisons across very different conditions (both fatal and non-fatal) that would otherwise not be readily comparable. A second objective was to provide a measurement method that could be used both to capture the state of global health and to guide policy decisions, particularly through the use of the measure in cost-effectiveness analyses (Murray 1996). Thus, the results from the project would allow us to identify the conditions that cause the greatest burden of disease across the world, providing important information for decisions about appropriate priorities for health interventions.

A central feature of the GBD is the metric in which disease burdens are expressed: the 'disability-adjusted life-year' (DALY). DALYs combine life-years lost due to premature mortality and years lived with certain disabilities or health conditions, weighted by the severity of the condition (Murray 1996; Lopez et al. 2006). For example, thirty DALYs could represent one person's loss of thirty fully healthy life-years, or her living for sixty years with a disability with a severity weight of 0.5. DALYs are also aggregated across individuals; for example, thirty DALYs could also represent thirty individuals losing one fully healthy year of life, or sixty individuals living for one year with a disability weighed at 0.5 for its severity.

First results from the GBD study, depicting the burden of disease in 1990, were published in 1996, followed by updates in subsequent years (World Health Organization 2002b; Mathers et al. 2008). The methodology of the GBD is currently being revised; the GBD 2010, expected to become available in 2012, will estimate the disease burden in 1990 and 2005 and provide projections for 2010.[2] Full details of the new methodology have yet to be published; one major change, however, that has already been announced concerns the derivation of disability weights, which I discuss briefly below.

The results of the GBD study are presented in vast tables listing DALYs lost, broken down by the health condition by which they are caused, or according to geographic region. The results indicate, for example, that non-communicable diseases, such as cancers, heart and cerebrovascular disease, are major contributors to the burden of disease across the world (Lopez et al. 2006). The GBD also brought attention to non-fatal conditions, such as neuropsychiatric conditions; in particular, unipolar depressive disorders have emerged as the third leading cause of the burden of disease worldwide (Mathers et al. 2008). DALYs have also been linked to specific risk factors such as various nutrient deficiencies, low fruit and vegetable intake, unprotected sex and urban air pollution (Ezzati et al. 2006).

Results from the GBD project can inform or influence policy in a number of different ways. Perhaps most prominently, the Disease Control Priorities Project, informed by GBD data, identifies appropriate priorities for global health interventions in developing countries (Jamison et al. 2006). This includes, for example, estimates of the cost-effectiveness of a host of different interventions in terms of DALYs averted per dollar spent. For example, voluntary testing and counselling to address HIV is estimated to cost between US$14 and US$261 per DALY averted, whereas antiretroviral treatment is estimated at US$350 to US$500 per DALY averted (Laxminarayan et al. 2006). This information is sometimes also expressed in terms of how many DALYs can be averted by US$1 million invested in particular treatments. For example, spending this sum on the provision of bypass surgery is estimated to avert fewer than forty DALYs; using this money to extend immunisation coverage with standard child vaccinations could avert 50,000 to 500,000 DALYs (Jamison 2006: 25). Such estimates can inform decisions among different types of interventions addressing a particular health condition (such as provision of free condoms versus education campaigns to prevent the spread of HIV), but also choices among interventions that address different conditions (such as free condoms to prevent the spread of HIV versus bed nets to prevent the spread of malaria, for example). One global health organisation, Population Services International (PSI), explicitly measures the impact of its work in terms of DALYs averted.[3] Information about the global disease burden has also been used to criticise the current allocation of global health aid, which remains focused on infectious diseases despite the finding that, even in low-income countries, the greatest burden of disease results from non-communicable disease (Stuckler et al. 2008). The GBD researchers have also used a measure similar to DALYs – health-adjusted life-expectancy (HALE) – to assess the performance of healthcare systems, and variation in HALE across individuals has been proposed as a measure of health inequality (Murray and Evans 2003).

THE 'NORMATIVE SHADOW' AND THE 'RESTRICTED INFORMATION REQUIREMENT'

As the GBD researchers explain, their project was meant to provide data that could inform global health policy. However, the inclusion of this objective appears to reflect not only the project's ambitions but also the recognition that any health measure would *inevitably* affect health policy (Murray 1996). Experience with indicators such as child mortality rates and the Human Development Index suggests that such measures are used by policy-makers, for example, to set policy goals and assess their performance against them. Thus, in developing health measures, we must take into account how such measures may come to be used in policy decisions and allow these considerations to affect the methodology on which the health measure is based. As Christopher Murray, one of the leading figures in the GBD project, explains:

if a measure is used, it will influence policy debate, permeate the thinking of decision-makers and become part of the culture of the subject. In other words, an indicator that is widely used will soon become normative through its use. The infant mortality rate, life expectancy and, to the extent they are adopted, DALYs, are used normatively and thus become normative measures. The normative aspects of indicators should be recognized clearly in the design of an indicator. This is not to suggest that the proponent of a new indicator bears responsibility for all intended or unintended uses of the measure *in perpetuo*. Rather, it is prudent to recognize the normative shadow that health measures cast and to try to reason carefully about their likely normative uses and the implications of such uses for the design of health indicators. (Murray 1996: 3)

Concerns about this 'normative shadow' have affected the GBD methodology in a number of respects. First, the particular health state valuation method used – the person trade-off – appears to have been chosen because it constructs disability weights from individuals' preferences about how health resources should be allocated between groups of individuals with different conditions. Second, if GBD data affect decisions, it is essential that we treat 'like as like' when evaluating the burden associated with particular health conditions; the only pieces of information affecting the measurement of the burden should be age and sex (the 'restricted information' requirement). Age and sex are reflected through the use of age-weighting and different life expectancies for men and women. Information that is *excluded* from the GBD measure includes differences in life expectancies in different countries as well as environmental factors that shape individuals' experience of particular health conditions.

DISABILITY WEIGHTS AND THE 'PERSON TRADE-OFF'

Central to health measurement – not just for DALYs but also for other health measures, such as quality-adjusted life-years (QALYs)[4] – is the ability to compare very different health states within a single 'currency'. This requires that 'disability weights' be attached to different health states so that time lived with that condition can be weighed accordingly. These disability weights, ranging from 0 to 1, express the deviation of a life-year lived in this state from a life-year lived in full health, with 0 being the weight attached to fully healthy life-years and higher numbers reflecting increasingly severe disabilities. It is only through the 'valuation' of different health states that information on non-fatal health experience and information on mortality can be combined into a single measure, making this a crucial element of health measures (Salomon et al. 2003).

Different methods exist for health state 'valuation', that is, the procedure through which disability weights are assigned to particular health conditions. Most of these methods ask individuals to respond to different hypothetical choice scenarios that involve different health conditions. For example, we might find out how many fully healthy years participants consider equivalent to a longer time period lived with a particular disability or disease. Disability weights can then be calculated from these responses.[5]

The disability weights of the original GBD study were based on the 'person trade-off' (PTO) method. Whereas other health valuation methods ask respondents to consider different scenarios in which they themselves experience certain health states, in the PTO respondents assume the perspective of a decision-maker who must choose among different interventions that prevent deaths or disease for different groups of individuals. Thus, as Murray notes, 'by its construction the PTO method appears to include some element of distributional preference in the estimated magnitude of health state preference' (Murray 1996: 29). Although this is somewhat ambiguous in the GBD researchers' own arguments, Nord (2002) suggests that PTO was used in the GBD methodology *precisely for this reason*: given that DALYs would be used in resource allocation decisions, disability weights that are influenced by distributional preferences were thought to be particularly suitable. The decision in favour of PTO over other health valuation methods thus seems to reflect the anticipated 'normative' use of the GBD data in resource allocation decisions.

One strand of criticism of the DALY focuses on the particular version of the PTO used for the GBD project. The GBD used two different PTO questions. The first asked respondents to consider a scenario in which they could either extend the lives of a certain number of healthy individuals or extend the lives of a certain number of individuals in a particular health state (PTO1). For instance, they have to choose between a) extending the lives of 1,000 healthy individuals for one year and b) extending the lives of 2,000 blind individuals for one year. In the second scenario (PTO2), participants choose between extending the lives of healthy people and curing individuals of the health state under consideration. For example, they may have to choose between a) extending the lives of 1,000 healthy individuals for one year or b) giving perfect vision to 2,000 blind individuals (who will live for one year subsequently) (see Murray 1996). With both questions, the number of individuals concerned is varied to the point where participants are indifferent between the two options. From these numbers, disability weights can be generated. For example, if respondents are indifferent between extending the lives of 1,000 non-disabled people for one year and extending the lives of 5,000 blind individuals (PTO1), then this would result in a disability weight of 0.8 (1 – [1000/5000]) (see Arnesen and Nord 1999). PTO1 and PTO2 were considered to be equivalent and participants had to resolve any inconsistencies in their responses to the two scenarios.

Critics, however, have argued that PTO1 and PTO2 are not in fact equivalent and that this version of the PTO implies that respondents should attach lesser value to saving the lives of disabled people than to saving the lives of non-disabled individuals (see Arnesen and Nord 1999). When considering PTO1, respondents may indicate that they do not wish to discriminate against disabled individuals by indicating indifference between a) and b) when the number of individuals in each is equal. This, however, would result in a disability weight of 0, implying that the disability in question is *no worse* than full health. Further, respondents had to resolve discrepancies in their responses to PTO1 and PTO2, implying that responses are inconsistent if participants do not discriminate between disabled and non-disabled individuals in PTO1. In addition to concerns about the judgements implicit in this methodology, the requirement that participants make their responses to PTO1 and PTO2 consistent with each other may skew the resulting disability weights (Arnesen and Nord 1999).

This is, of course, a significant worry about the original GBD methodology. (The discrepancies between disability weights generated from PTO1 and PTO2 vary by condition; see Murray 1996: 39 for details.) It should be noted, however, that in more recent work, the GBD researchers used variants of PTO2 to describe the person trade-off method (for example, Salomon and Murray 2004). For the forthcoming GBD 2010 study, PTO has been abandoned completely for a different valuation method, as I explain in more detail below. Most significant for present purposes is the fact that PTO seems to have been chosen in part because it is influenced by respondents' distributive preferences, with a view to the influence that GBD data is likely to have on resource allocation decisions.

DALYS AND THE 'RESTRICTED INFORMATION' REQUIREMENT

One implication of the 'normative shadow' is the GBD researchers' insistence that only age and sex should affect the calculation of the burden of disease. This section begins by discussing how age and sex are taken into account in constructing DALYs, particularly in relation to the use of age-weights and different life-expectancy standards for men and women. I then go on to discuss two elements that are explicitly excluded from affecting DALY measurements: differences in life expectancy across countries and the effects of contextual factors on individuals' experience of health states. These methodological decisions reflect, in different ways, concerns about the role of GBD results in policy decisions.

Age-weighting

DALYs lost due to premature mortality are calculated as the shortfall from a specified life expectancy. A death at an early age would lead to more life-years – and therefore more DALYs – lost than a death at a later age. However, controversially, the GBD project also applied non-uniform age-weights in its calculations, giving lower weights to DALYs lost in children and older adults. To illustrate the impact of age-weighting in the standard DALY, Arnesen and Kapiriri calculate that the number of DALYs lost would be equal if 185 newborns, seventeen 6-month-olds, five 2-year-olds, one 25-year-old, two 67-year-olds or three 83-year-olds suffered the same condition for one month (Arnesen and Kapiriri 2004).

Two explanations for this move appear in the original exposition of the GBD methodology. First, empirical studies suggest that people prefer to save lives of young adults over young children, and those of young over older adults; this motivates Murray to incorporate age-weights into the GBD. Second, these preferences can be seen as reflecting the different 'social value' of different life stages, as both children and old adults are dependent on young and middle-aged adults (Murray 1996: 55; Murray 1994: 434–5). While this move has been criticised (for example, Bognar 2008), it appears to be based on the idea that the GBD approach should cohere with people's preferences about distributions of health benefits across individuals at different ages;

this move, then, again reflects concerns about the role of GBD data in resource allocation decisions.

Male vs Female Life Expectancy

The second factor that DALYs are supposed to reflect is sex. In calculating how many life-years have been lost due to a particular disease, we have to decide what we consider the full life expectancy from which shortfalls can be calculated. In the vast majority of countries, women tend to live longer, on average, than men. To what extent, if at all, should this difference be reflected in our health measure?

For the original GBD study, Murray argued that DALYs should reflect that portion of the difference between male and female life expectancy that is the result of biological or genetic rather than behavioural or environmental factors. The GBD researchers estimated this difference to be 2.5 years, that is, 4.5 years less than the *actual* life expectancy gap of around seven years (Murray 1996). At the same time, however, the GBD researchers suggest that this approach is open to challenge on equity grounds, as 'a male death at age 40 should count as the same duration of life lost as a female death at age 40' (Murray 1996: 17), and that future revisions of the GBD may use the same life expectancy for both men and women.

It is not clear why the GBD researchers chose to integrate an estimate of the biologically determined differences in life expectancy in their measure if they believed this move to be open to challenge. One consideration Murray mentions is that, while it is not currently possible to redress such biological differences directly, they may become amenable to interventions in the future. These concerns are reminiscent of Margaret Whitehead's approach to health inequality, which has been highly influential in the global health context. She suggests that health disparities due to natural or biological variation would not generally be regarded as unjust; further, health disparities can be unjust only if they were avoidable (Whitehead 1991). Murray's willingness to adapt this aspect of the GBD methodology in the future may then be based on the assumption that once technological progress makes even the biologically determined portion of the survival gap amenable to intervention, it would be *unfair* not to set the same life expectancy standard for both men and women. Importantly, even if amenability is a criterion in assessing the unfairness of inequalities,[6] it seems irrelevant when calculating how many life-years were lost when someone dies at a particular age. If it is indeed such concerns that shaped the GBD methodology at this point, this aspect of the DALY too reflects concerns about the 'normative shadow' of health measures.

Ideal Standard of Life Expectancy

A further issue in choosing appropriate life expectancies to calculate life-years lost is whether they should reflect the vast disparities in average life expectancies that we find across the world. Following the 'restrictive information' principle, the GBD uses a 'hypothetical norm' (Michaud et al. 2001: 535), or an 'ideal standard' (Murray 1996: 14), of life expectancy to calculate the number of life-years lost, irrespective of local life expectancies. The GBD study relies on a single life expectancy (82.5 years for women, 80 years for men), irrespective of where a premature death occurs.

As critics have pointed out (for example, Williams 1999) – and as the GBD researchers fully acknowledge (Murray and Lopez 2000) – this move is motivated by concerns about equality:

> We articulate a principle of treating like health outcomes as like. For example, the premature death of a 40-year-old woman should contribute equally to estimates of the global burden of disease irrespective of whether she lives in the slums of Bogota or a wealthy suburb of Boston. [. . .] Community-specific characteristics such as local levels of mortality should not change the assumptions incorporated into the indicator design. (Murray 1994: 431)

The adoption of a single, 'aspirational' (Williams 2000: 85) life expectancy was to ensure that 'deaths at the same age in all communities contribute equally to the burden of disease so that like outcomes are treated as like' (Murray 1996: 16). Again, the underlying concern is to ensure that the use of DALYs in decision-making does not generate unfairness, even if – as critics have argued – this could make the DALY a less accurate measure of the disease burden across countries. The use of a single life expectancy means that when, say, a 30-year-old in a wealthy country dies of cancer, this leads to the same loss of DALYs as the cancer death of a 30-year-old in a poor country, even though average life expectancies in those countries would suggest that, without the cancer, the former would have gone on to live for a greater number of years than the former. Designing a health measure such that both deaths lead to the same DALY loss arguably leads to distortions because the number of life-years lost *due to the cancer* are not, in fact, the same. Instead, 'the burden that is measured by DALYs is the burden of disease and underdevelopment, and not that of disease alone' (Anand and Hanson 1997: 690).

Context: 'Disability' vs 'Handicap'

A further, important implication of the 'restricted information' requirement is that information about the context in which individuals live should not affect the measurement of the burden associated with their conditions. In the terminology of the WHO's *International Classification of Impairments, Disabilities and Handicaps* (ICIDH), to which the early GBD work refers, DALYs should capture disability (for example, loss of motor function) not handicaps (that is, the impact of the disability on the individual, given her particular social context) (Murray 1996: 33).

The GBD researchers emphasise that health must be kept conceptually distinct from its effects on other, more subjective concepts, such as utility, quality of life or well-being, many of which are mediated by the environments in which people live (for example, Chatterji et al. 2002; Salomon et al. 2003). A health metric that would allow for environments to influence our assessment of disease burdens would have the counter-intuitive result that individuals become 'healthier' as a result of environmental changes that make a particular condition less burdensome; health should be regarded as an 'attribute of individuals rather than environments' (Salomon et al. 2003: 304).

In addition to these conceptual arguments, however, this move also again reflects fairness considerations. Murray notes that 'allocating resources to avert handicap as opposed to disability could exacerbate inequalities' (Murray 1996: 33). A cognitive impairment, for example, would be less of a disadvantage for those living in a remote rural community than for those living in urban areas:

Pursuing handicap could, and probably would, lead us to invest in avoiding mental retardation in the rich and well educated but not in the poor. To avoid the obvious problems with such an approach, one must focus on disability rather than handicap. (Murray 1996: 33)

This aspect of the GBD methodology has been criticised heavily. One major concern is that, despite the GBD researchers' arguments, this move actually contributes to *in*equality. In the global context, the implications of living in countries with different income levels or levels of development is particularly salient. Allotey et al. (2003) illustrate the importance of this point by exploring the vast discrepancies in the effects of paraplegia on individuals in Cameroon compared to Australia. In Cameroon, paraplegics suffer serious, sometimes even fatal, pressure sores; they may not have access to a wheelchair; they may not be able to maintain personal hygiene because they lack access to running water; they may become isolated from their communities. Allotey et al. argue that there is a 'development gradient': the severity of living with a particular health condition decreases the more developed the country is. Thus, the use of DALYs as they are constructed within the GBD study could exacerbate health inequalities between low- and high-income countries, as the GBD methodology underestimates the disease burden in less developed areas (Allotey et al. 2003). This concern has led some to argue that the disability weights attached to particular health states should vary depending on environmental and developmental differences between countries (Reidpath et al. 2003).

The concern, then, both among GBD researchers and their critics, has been that our health measure should not disadvantage those in less developed communities vis-à-vis citizens of wealthier countries. Despite disagreement about the effects of excluding contextual factors from DALY calculations (Murray focusing on a condition that would be *less* burdensome in low-income countries, critics on conditions that would be *more* burdensome), implicit in this debate is again the concern that health measures must not contribute or lead to unfair policy decisions and that the underlying methodology should be designed to avoid such effects.

FAIRNESS CONSIDERATIONS IMPLICIT IN THE GBD: DOES IT MATTER?

The previous sections illustrated various aspects of the GBD methodology that were influenced by concerns about the 'normative shadow', that is, the ways in which health measures might influence health policy. Through the 'restricted information' requirement, the DALY methodology aims to exclude considerations that should not affect resource allocation decisions. This section begins by discussing the conceptual problems raised when the methodology used to derive health measures reflects considerations of fairness. From a more practical perspective, however, the limitations of available health measurement methods blur this conceptual distinction and, it has been argued, there may be good pragmatic reasons for not insisting on conceptual clarity in this case.

Murray argues for the 'restricted information' requirement with the following scenario:

> Imagine a situation where two patients arrive at an emergency room both in a coma from meningitis, but there is only enough antibiotic to treat one of them. The two patients are totally identical in every respect except that one is rich and the other is poor. [. . .] I argue through the restricted information proposition that we should be completely indifferent to treating one over the other. The income of the patients has no bearing on who should receive the life-saving intervention. (Murray 1996: 7)

Similarly, in response to the suggestion that individual characteristics, such as a person's ability to adapt to a particular condition, should be reflected in burden of disease calculations, he argues:

> the notion that we should count a given health outcome [. . .] as more important in an individual who has a lower capacity to adapt psychologically than in an individual who has a higher capacity to adapt psychologically would appear to be manifestly unfair. (Murray 1996: 7)

Thus, he concludes, DALYs have a 'strongly egalitarian flavor' (Murray 1996: 7).

However, critics have challenged this line of argument: it does not follow from the fact that a particular criterion ought not be relevant in health resource allocation decisions that this criterion should not be relevant in health *measurement* (Bognar 2008; Broome 2002). Rather, Broome argues, examples such as these show that claims about fairness

must be kept distinct from claims about 'goodness', that is, the good
done by reducing disease. Maximising a desired outcome such as
health or goodness may lead us to choose one patient over the other;
this consideration, however, is outweighed by fairness, which requires
us to be impartial between the two patients: 'Once we see that fairness
is a distinct consideration from goodness, we will not need to try and
incorporate considerations of fairness into our measure of goodness';
allowing fairness considerations to influence our health measure in the
way implicit in the GBD approach 'distorts' our measurement (Broome
2002: 99).

How significant are these conceptual worries in the context of the
GBD? In practice, the limitations of available measurement instruments may lead to various deviations from the 'information restriction'
requirement. In deriving disability weights, for example, respondents
in the original GBD study were asked to assume that health conditions were affecting individuals living in the 'average social response or
milieu' (Murray 1996: 38). Thus, preferences about health states reflect
assumptions about the environment and about how this environment
interacts with health states to affect individuals. Murray admits that
this allows for some ambiguity within the GBD approach with respect
to whether what is actually measured is 'disability' or 'handicap'.
Although the GBD aims to measure disability rather than handicap,
what its methods *actually* capture is a 'construct somewhere between
disability and handicap', or an 'average level of handicap' (Murray
1996: 33–4). Preferences among different health states will also reflect a
host of other considerations that affect how 'bad' respondents perceive
a particular condition to be. For example, disability weights seem to be
somewhat higher when respondents believe that a condition is subject
to stigmatisation (Üstün et al. 1999).

There may also be pragmatic reasons to tread carefully in distinguishing fairness and goodness in defining DALYs, given the context
in which such measures are employed. Brock explains:

A measure that seems to have the evident and straightforward
implication that saving lives and, for example, preventing AIDS
in developing countries does less good and has less value than
doing so in developed countries – that the lives of the rich are of
more value than those of the poor – would obviously be subject to
and would no doubt receive serious attack in political and policy

contexts. Insisting that although the good produced by saving a life in the developing world is indeed less than in the developed world, on grounds of fairness we do not want to give priority to the latter over the former, might do little to deflect that attack in a world marked by deep sensitivity and suspicion by many in the developing countries about inadequate concern in the developed countries for them and their problems. If there are good reasons of fairness, and perhaps other reasons as well, for ignoring other non-health differences in the goodness of lives across countries, pragmatic policy or political considerations may support not strictly separating all fairness concerns from the burden of disease measure. (Brock 2002: 119)

In designing health measures, researchers must determine how and to what extent, if at all, such considerations should influence the methodology adopted.

THE GBD AND HEALTH POLICY

The previous sections outlined how the GBD study has been shaped by concerns about how its results would influence global health policy. This, the critics argue, distorts the data gained from the project. Further, the assumptions implicit in DALY measurements are not necessarily uncontroversial. For example, age-weights, which were included in the GBD study to reflect 'social preferences' for resource allocation among individuals in different age groups, may well be considered unfair.

Moreover, DALYs cannot capture, and may even mask, fairness considerations that will be highly relevant when making policy decisions. For example, policy-makers may be interested in pursuing not just the improvement of health but also the reduction of health inequalities; again, such considerations are not reflected in DALY measures. Furthermore, we may want to give some priority to those with the most severe conditions. However, since DALYs are aggregated across individuals, it is not clear to what extent a certain number of DALYs reflects the severity of a particular condition rather than its prevalence (Arnesen and Kapiriri 2004). A high number of DALYs can result from a mild but very common condition or from a rarer but very severe disease. Advocates of the GBD project can respond that their aim is to provide a summary measure of health and that the severity of particular diseases can be gauged from descriptions of the health states in question. It should be noted, however, that at least some presentations of GBD results lend themselves to less nuanced interpretations of the data. For example, when considering lists of the costs of different policy interventions in terms of DALYs averted per dollar spent, policy-makers may be tempted to focus on those interventions that promise the most 'value for money', rather than evaluating the data in the context of other relevant considerations.

Some commentators have suggested that such considerations could, to some extent, be integrated into health measures. For example, Nord and colleagues propose that health measures be coupled with weights that reflect the priority that those with the most severe conditions should receive. These weights would be based on estimates of the population's preferences about distributions; the measure would then be more accurately described as a measure of 'health-related societal value' (Nord et al. 1999; see also Nord 2002). Similarly, Williams suggests that health measures could be combined with weights that reflect concerns about intergenerational equity (Williams 1997). Such weighted measures could provide a more appropriate tool for policy-makers in that they integrate a broader range of relevant considerations; policies that try to minimise these weighted DALYs then automatically give some weight to such concerns.

Other critics of the GBD have recommended a very different approach, arguing that the normative assumptions of the GBD data should be made as transparent as possible, by presenting information on disability weights, age groups affected by particular conditions and their prevalence separately, rather than aggregating all this information within DALYs (Arnesen and Kapiriri 2004).

While the GBD study is unlikely to go as far as Arnesen and Kapiriri recommend, recent developments suggest that the project has begun to change its stance on how best to respond to the 'normative shadow'. There now appears to be a clearer focus on providing an accurate measure of the burden of disease and a greater emphasis on the limitations of the role that such a measure can play in policy decisions.

With respect to health state valuation, recent work by GBD researchers emphasises that commonly used valuation methods elicit preferences not just about health but also about other factors (in the case of the PTO, preferences about distributions), and that while this may be appropriate for certain contexts, it is undesirable when aiming to provide a measure that allows comparisons of health levels in different populations (Salomon and Murray 2004). In fact, rather than relying on disability weights derived from PTO, the forthcoming GBD 2010 will apply a new method, which asks respondents to indicate which of two individuals in different health states is 'healthier than' the other; disability weights are then derived from the results of these pairwise comparisons (Salomon 2010). This suggests that instead of allowing distributive preferences to affect disability weights, the focus is on the relative severity of different health conditions.

In recent publications, the GBD researchers have also been more explicit about the limitations of DALYs in informing policy decisions. Murray et al. note that:

> Many authors have rightly focused on a range of values relevant to the allocation of scarce resources that may enhance individuals' health. However, many of these considerations bring us far from the common-sense statement that one population is healthier than another. At least for the purposes of comparative statements on health it may be necessary to distance the development of summary measures from the complex values that have to be considered in the allocation of scarce resources. In other words, we can quite reasonably choose to measure population health in one way and conclude that scarce resources should not be allocated strictly to maximize population health as so measured. (Murray, Salomon and Mathers 2000: 986, references omitted)

GBD data are now also commonly presented with different versions of the DALY (for example, with uniform and non-uniform age-weights) and sensitivity analyses are provided to determine the effects of particular elements of the methodology on the overall results. This enhances the transparency of GBD data and gives users greater discretion over which aspects of the GBD methodology they wish to accept and which elements they find problematic.

CONCLUSION

Results from the GBD study have been prominent in global health. The GBD study aims to provide a systematic and objective assessment of the global burden of ill-health and the contributions of different conditions and risk factors to that burden. As I highlight in this chapter, the DALY methodology was designed with the influence of health measures on health policy in mind: DALYs should not lead to unfair policy decisions, particularly in relation to health priorities and resource allocation. Critics have been concerned that allowing concerns about fairness to shape what is supposed to be a measure of health is conceptually flawed and could distort the results obtained from the project. Recent revisions of the GBD methodology suggest a greater emphasis on the primary role of DALYs as a measure of the burden of disease and the limitations that must be borne in mind when using GBD data in policy decisions. These developments may lead to a more accurate description of global health but they also place a greater burden on policy-makers to find an appropriate role for GBD data in their decisions.

Notes

1. I would like to thank Sam Harper, Nicholas King, Patti Lenard, Christine Straehle and Garrath Williams for helpful comments on earlier drafts of this paper.
2. See www.globalburden.org; http://www.who.int/healthinfo/global_burden_disease/en/.
3. See www.psi.org.
4. The underlying principle of adjusting life-years depending on disability is similar to the construction of quality-adjusted life-years (QALYs). However, while QALYs express health *gains*, DALYs represent health *losses*. 1 QALY represents one life-year lived in full health, while 1 DALY represents one fully healthy life-year lost.
5. For an account of different health valuation methods and their implications, see, for example, Salomon and Murray (2004).
6. Norheim and Asada (2009) suggest an argument along these lines. However, others have argued that the avoidability or amenability of particular health inequalities should not affect our assessment of whether or not such inequalities are *unfair*; see, for example, Braveman and Gruskin (2003) and Segall (2009). Segall explicitly challenges the idea that differences in male and female life expectancy are not unfair.

Chapter 9

EXPLORING A SUFFICIENCY VIEW OF HEALTH EQUITY[1]

Yukiko Asada

1. INTRODUCTION

Health inequality or, more precisely, health *inequity* – morally problematic health inequality – has remained an important issue in many
countries over the past few decades and recently became increasingly so in the global context (Segall 2009; Wikler and Brock 2007).
Epidemiologists and public and population health researchers have
documented numerous health inequalities and inequities within and
across populations (Harper et al. 2007; James et al. 2007; Smits and
Monden 2009; World Health Organization 2000). Over the years, many
concerted efforts to reduce health inequities have emerged nationally and internationally, most notably the World Health Organization
(WHO)'s Commission on Social Determinants of Health (2008). Among
a profusion of academic and policy inquiries of health inequities, one
of the most important recent developments is serious philosophical investigation into how to define health inequity. Informed by the
literature suggesting the importance of social determinants of health,
philosophers no longer consider illness as bad luck but regard the distribution of health as an issue of justice and fairness. Philosophically
oriented scholars thus began to provide rich accounts of when health
inequalities become of moral concern and why we should be morally
concerned about some health inequalities (Daniels 2008; Hausman
2009; Marchand, Wikler and Landesman 1998; Segall 2009). These are
important questions to be clear about. Without knowing what exactly
we wish to reduce and articulating why we wish to do so, how can we
begin the work and ask others to join the force?

To determine which health inequalities are morally problematic,
most serious philosophical investigation, to date, has focused on *causes*

of health inequalities. An underlying premise in such investigation is that health inequalities due to all causes are not of moral concern – only those due to certain factors are. Health inequalities caused by, for example, chance events (for example, being hit by lightning), personal choices (fully informed free decision to sky dive) or demographic factors (death at an old age) are often considered to be morally acceptable (Asada 2007). Various definitions of health inequity currently offered in the literature are born out of disagreements regarding which causes are, using an increasingly popular terminology, 'legitimate' (leading to morally permissible health inequalities) or 'illegitimate' (leading to health inequities) (Fleurbaey and Schokkaert 2009).

In this chapter, I explore an alternative approach to defining health inequity. I propose a sufficiency view of health equity that states, briefly, society should be concerned about whether each person satisfies a sufficient level of health regardless of cause. In addition, using poverty analysis as a methodological foundation, I demonstrate how the proposed sufficiency view of health equity can be used as a basis for empirical analysis. I argue that a sufficiency view of health can supplement, rather than replace, current health inequity perspectives and analyses. This is because people with myriad differing perspectives of health inequity would still find the information on insufficient health useful (just as information on poverty and income inequality enriches the other and co-exists in the sphere of income distribution). The plan of this chapter is as follows. Section 2 introduces a sufficiency view of health inequity and focuses on the conceptual issues. Section 3 provides an empirical demonstration based on a sufficiency view of health equity using the 2002–3 Joint Canada–United States Survey of Health. Section 4 concludes with discussing issues for further development.

2. THE CONCEPT

In the past decade, serious philosophical examination of definitions of health inequities has emerged (Anand, Peter and Sen 2006; Daniels 2008; Powers and Faden 2008; Ruger 2010; Segall 2009). It suggests that socio-economic status-related health inequity, the most studied health inequity, is only but one definition of health inequity among many other possibilities. For example, one definition of health inequity, keenly debated in recent years, is equal opportunity for health (Segall 2009; Le Grand 1991; Rosa Dias 2009; Whitehead 1992). In its essence, equal opportunity for health means ensuring that all members of society have equal opportunities to be healthy. Scholars formulate the notion of equal opportunity for health differently, but one formulation offered by Segall argues, 'It is unjust for individuals to be worse off than others due to outcomes that it would have been unreasonable to expect them to avoid' (Segall 2009: 13). Central to this view is the notion of individual responsibility for health.[2] This perspective considers that health inequalities due to factors beyond individual control are unfair while those due to factors under individual control are not. Another example of health inequity perspective, often implicitly suggested in the empirical health inequity literature, is policy amenability, which holds that health inequities are those resulting from situations where society could have intervened but did not (Asada and Hedemann 2002; Norheim and Asada 2009).

Fleurbaey and Schokkaert recently proposed a model to unite various popular views of health inequities and bridge the concepts to empirical investigation (Fleurbaey and Schokkaert 2009). The premise of their model is that one needs to examine *causes* of health inequalities to define health inequities. In their words, some causes have 'legitimate' (or ethically justifiable or unproblematic) influence on a person's health state, and others have 'illegitimate' (or ethically unjustifiable or problematic) influence. Health inequalities caused by illegitimate factors are unfair or inequitable. They suggest that diverse definitions of health inequities derive from the disagreement regarding the legitimate–illegitimate distinction. For example, according to the aforementioned view of equal opportunity for health, one may consider health behaviours, such as smoking and physical activity, as largely individual preferences (thus, legitimate causes of health inequalities), while according to the view of policy amenability, one may regard these health behaviours as amenable to policy (hence, illegitimate).

While defining health inequities by examining causes of health inequalities is vastly popular, this is not the only way to define health inequities. Rather than examining causes, one can define health inequities by focusing on the *level* of health (Asada 2007). Or to put it more fully, one can consider strict equal health for all as the starting point in defining health inequity. Strict equal health, however, is not necessarily a morally attractive view as it denies personal choice too strongly and may demand levelling down of the healthy (Norheim and Asada 2009). If not strict equal health, then, what is the morally attractive distribution of health? To examine this question, one approach is to focus on causes of health inequalities and make the legitimate–illegitimate distinction of those causes. Another approach is to focus on the level of health and consider all causes of health inequalities as illegitimate.

An appeal to this latter approach, which I shall call a sufficiency view of health inequity, can be found in Elizabeth Anderson's critique of the recent trend in philosophical discussion regarding egalitarianism (more specifically, luck egalitarianism) (Anderson 1999). She believes that examining how people obtained certain essential resources in life and how they should be compensated for undeserved bad luck does not show respect to persons, a fundamental reason why we care about equality among people to begin with. She states, 'what citizens ultimately owe one another is the social conditions of freedoms people need to function as equal citizens' (Anderson 1999: 320).[3] Such social conditions may consist of a variety of spheres, including health. Society would then be concerned about whether each person satisfies a sufficient level of health regardless of how each person obtained a certain level of health.

To defend a sufficiency view of health, one must show the importance of health and justify why every person's health should satisfy at least the sufficient level. To argue for the importance of health, one needs to examine what good health is from an egalitarian perspective. A good starting point may be to characterise health by borrowing a framework of the long-standing egalitarian discussion regarding what to equalise: should we consider health as welfare (that is, well-being of each person), a resource (a good that every person wants regardless of his or her goal of life, such as political liberty and income) or a capability (a freedom each person earned from obtaining an important good) (Hausman and McPherson 2006)? As I describe below, considering health as a capability appears to offer the most fitting foundation for a sufficiency view of health.

Amartya Sen and Martha Nussbaum proposed to equalise capabilities, rather than welfare or resources (Nussbaum 2011; Sen 1992). Their approach considering capabilities as the focal point of egalitarianism is commonly known as the capabilities approach, and emerged from their frustration with welfarist and resourcist views. For Sen and Nussbaum, equalising welfare is too much (as society should not be responsible for what people freely choose to do in their lives) while equalising resources is not enough (as doing so does not adequately acknowledge diversity in internal characteristics among people). Simply providing the same resources does not lead to the same level of freedom in life. The proper focus of egalitarians, they argue, is not what people actually do and are ('functionings' such as reading and writing) but what people can do ('capabilities' such as literacy).

Sen and Nussbaum have different perspectives on how health may fit into the capabilities approach. Sen is deliberately ambiguous about what constitutes capabilities and only goes so far as to acknowledge that each individual should have an 'equivalent' capability set. Nussbaum, on the other hand, provides a list of ten central capabilities, including life ('being able to live to the end of a human life of normal length; not dying prematurely, or before one's life is so reduced as to be not worth living') and bodily health ('being able to have good health, including reproductive health; to be adequately nourished; to have adequate shelter') (Nussbaum 2011: 33). It is thus Nussbaum's version of the capabilities approach that can be applied to health most directly.

The capabilities approach implies the basic minimum (sufficient level) that society ought to ensure for its citizens. Nussbaum considers the basic minimum as a 'reference to an idea of human worth or dignity', instead of the literal interpretation suggesting that below the minimum people are better off if dead (Nussbaum 2000: 73). Extended, one might argue that persons are not allowed to make trade-offs between capabilities because, according to the capabilities approach, the sufficient level of each capability is vital for human worth or dignity. Above the sufficient level, however, depending on preferences and conceptions of good life, persons can trade-off capabilities. A sufficiency view of health inequity would then suggest that health inequalities below the sufficiency level are of moral concern but those above it are not.

An obvious question for a sufficiency view of health or, in fact, any other important good is whether it can serve as a complete distributional theory given that it is only concerned about the part of the distribution below a threshold. My answer to this question is pragmatic. Even if some regarded it as an incomplete perspective, they would not deny its usefulness at least as supplementary information to conventional views of health inequity considering the entire distribution of health. An analogy to the literature on income inequality and poverty might be helpful here. The literatures on income inequality (examining the entire distribution of income) and poverty (examining the part of the distribution of income below a threshold) co-exist without claiming

superiority to each other. Similarly, there is no reason to choose
between health inequity (based on the entire distribution) and insufficient health. A sufficiency view of health equity can enrich the field of
health inequity in a similar way as the literature on poverty does to that
of income inequality.

One of the most serious challenges of a sufficiency view of health
equity is defining sufficient health. This is particularly important in
applying the concept to empirical investigation. Here I briefly discuss
two inter-related issues that make this task challenging: universality
and infeasibility. First, when defining sufficient health, we must determine how universal it should be; more precisely, whether we wish to
focus on the same aspects of health and define the same level of sufficient health across all societies we are going to examine. Health is
multi-dimensional, and some societies might value certain aspects of
health more than others (for example, infertility is likely considered
more of an issue in India than in Canada). A further difficulty in defining health is distinctions between 'bare' health (for example, mobility
with paralysed legs) and 'bare' health with medical technologies (with
regenerative medicine), with non-human aids (with a wheelchair),
with human assistance (with a personal attendant), and/or with accommodating environmental factors (in a barrier-free built environment)
(Asada 2005). Paraplegia would be a more difficult condition in a society
with less advanced medicine or with less spirit of mutual co-operation.
Even if we agreed on what aspects of health we examine, the question
would remain as to how to set the level of sufficient health. Should the
level of sufficient health be the same for, for example, Canada a century
ago and now, or for contemporary Canada and Zimbabwe (the sickest
country in terms of age standardised disability-adjusted life-years in
2004 [World Health Organization 2004])?

What is at issue here is universality in relation to variation in
technological levels and cultures across societies. The technological
advancement of societies influences their overall level of health and
the availability of medical technologies and non-human aids. Cultural
values of societies affect the concept of health, the provision of human
assistance and accommodating environmental factors, and even the
overall level of health through some social determinants of health, such
as social capital. While the capabilities approach certainly implies universality, what it means is unclear at the level of specification required
for empirical investigation. For example, the widely used Human

Development Index (United Nations Development Programme 2010), which is broadly based on the capabilities approach, applies an almost, but not precisely, universal norm. It measures shortfalls from the norm set by the best and worst performances among the countries in the particular year of the assessment. The norm is thus universal across countries but not across time. Of course, any empirical application of concepts requires considerations for pragmatism and data availability. Nonetheless, specific questions of universality that empirical applications bring back to the concept of a sufficiency view of health equity may further enrich the concept itself.

Infeasibility is another difficulty when defining sufficient health. If societies were serious about a sufficiency view of health equity, they would go bankrupt. In some cases it would be prohibitively expensive to bring everyone to the sufficient level of health. The concern for costs is not limited to a sufficiency view of health equity but also applies to many other views. And one could reasonably argue that the cost consideration is not a question of health equity. In real world decision-making, one would need to balance multiple ideals, such as equity versus efficiency.

A real infeasibility challenge for a sufficiency view of health equity is the problem of the 'hopelessly sick'. However we define sufficient health, there will always be someone who cannot satisfy it. Note that we are not concerned about imprudence of the hopelessly sick that might have caused health below the sufficient level. The causal pathway does not matter in a sufficiency view of health equity. Rather, the problem of the hopelessly sick results from inadequate medical technology and knowledge. Even without resource constraint, there will be an occasion when medical technology and knowledge currently available are not enough to bring every person's health up to the sufficient level. One solution might be to add a conditional clause to the definition of sufficient health, such as 'as long as technologically feasible'. However, this quickly opens up a question related to the universality challenge above. Should we decide to accept technological limitation here, then we should acknowledge differences in technological advancement when defining sufficient health in different societies. Another solution might be to consider compensation from other spheres of capabilities, but this procedure obviously violates a fundamental aspect of a sufficiency view of health equity: that persons are not allowed to make trade-offs between spheres below the sufficiency level.

3. EMPIRICAL DEMONSTRATION

In this section, I explore empirical applications of a sufficiency view of health. The primary purpose of the analysis presented below is to show the process of bridging the concept and empirical analysis rather than to highlight results of the analysis. Specifically, I aim to underscore the role of the poverty literature as a rich methodological foundation for measuring inequity from a perspective of sufficient health. In addition, I aim to suggest one pragmatic strategy to operationalise a definition of sufficient health that is cognisant of the universality and infeasibility discussion above.

3.1 Methods

Data

Data for the empirical application of a sufficiency view of health equity come from the Joint Canada/United States Survey of Health (JCUSH), a cross-sectional population health survey jointly conducted by Statistics Canada and the US National Center for Health Statistics in 2002–3 (Statistics Canada and United States National Center for Health Statistics 2004). The target population was non-institutionalised Canadian and US household residents aged eighteen and older. The JCUSH questionnaire included questions regarding health status, health behaviour, socio-economic status, healthcare utilisation and health insurance status. The sample sizes for this analysis are 2,891 (Canada) and 3,798 (US).[4,5]

Measure of Health – The Health Utilities Index

The measurement of health for this analysis is the Health Utilities Index Mark 3 (HUI), a generic (that is, not disease-specific) health-related quality of life measure. The HUI was developed by researchers at McMaster University and is widely used in Canada and internationally (Horsman et al. 2003). The HUI measures the respondent's functional levels in eight dimensions (vision, hearing, speech, mobility, dexterity, emotion, cognition and pain) and converts the respondent's functional levels into a score based on social preferences over health states. For example, the HUI score for a near-sighted but otherwise fully functional individual is 0.973, and this score reflects the average societal preference, rather than the respondent's assessment, of how good this particular health state is compared to full health. Though the preferences were obtained from a somewhat limited sample (a sample of the community dwelling population in Hamilton, Ontario), they have extensively been assessed and are now accepted for national and international use (Furlong et al. 1998). The HUI scores for health states range from −0.360 to 1.000 on a scale in which 0.000 represents dead, and 1.000 represents perfect health. Negative scores mean health states worse than dead. A difference of 0.030 or greater is considered to be clinically meaningful (Drummond 2001; Grootendorst, Feeny and Furlong 2000).

Health-related quality of life measures, such as the HUI, are well suited for an empirical application of a sufficiency view of health equity. In Section 2, I argued that the understanding of health as a capability supports a sufficiency view of health. What many health-related quality of life measures attempt to measure happens to come close to the concept of a capability. Most health-related quality of life measures assess function levels rather than particular diseases. The choice of dimensions of function differs by different instruments, for example, vision, hearing, speech, mobility, dexterity, emotion, cognition and pain in the HUI, but mobility, self-care, usual activities, pain/discomfort and anxiety/depression in EQ-5D, another widely used health-related quality of life measure (Kind, Brooks and Rabin 2005). The function that most health-related quality of life measures assess (for example, being able to move around without a cane or other assistance) can be considered as an enabler of what each person wishes to do (such as, for example, running). Thus, despite the confusing terminologies – 'function' used in health-related quality of life measures and 'functioning' used in the capabilities approach – the function captured by most health-related quality of life measures is a capability.

Sufficient Health
In this study, I define the sufficient level of health as the average HUI in each age group (18–44, 45–64 and 65+ years). This measurement decision implies an agreement on the definition of health across societies but acknowledges a need for adjustments of the sufficient level according to the technological advancement, available knowledge and resource constraint in each society. More specifically, the use of the HUI in both countries acknowledges that they both value the same aspects of health that the HUI measures. Focusing on the average HUI

in each country means that the sufficient level is set at the level which society can reasonably provide to its people given the technological advancement, available knowledge and resource constraint in each society. Setting the sufficient level differently to different age groups acknowledges the influence of the general biological ageing process on health and the lack of the current medical knowledge and technology to reverse such process. In short, sufficient health in this study is partially universal and attempts to address the infeasibility problem.

Measure of Health Inequity: The Foster-Greer-Thorbecke (FGT) Measure
From a measurement perspective, a sufficiency view of health equity resembles analyses of poverty. In both cases, the concept of a threshold plays a central role in the measurement. Following the poverty literature, it is possible to measure insufficient health by focusing on the following three characteristics (Sen 1997a):

The head count
The health gap
The distribution of health below the sufficient level

By the head count, we can assess the proportion of people below the level of sufficient health (Figure 9.1a). By the health gap, we can evaluate the depth of insufficient health, in other words, how far off people are from sufficient health (Figure 9.1b). Furthermore, we can consider the distribution of insufficient health (Figure 9.1c). These characteristics offer richer descriptions of insufficient health in an increasing order, and it is desirable to capture all three characteristics.

In this study I employ one of the widely used poverty measures assessing all of these three characteristics, the Foster-Greer-Thorbecke (FGT) measure (Sen 1997a), as the measure of health inequity based on a sufficiency view. Specifically, the FGT measure captures these three characteristics by changing the value of a parameter α. When $\alpha=0$, the FGT measure calculates the head count; when $\alpha=1$, it estimates the health gap; and when $\alpha=2$, it assesses all three characteristics including the distribution of insufficient health. Regardless of the value of α, the FGT measure takes values between 0 and 1. Zero means that everybody satisfies sufficient health, and a greater FGT value indicates a greater head count (for FGT $[\alpha=0]$), health gap (for FGT $[\alpha=1]$) or inequity (for FGT $[\alpha=2]$).[6]

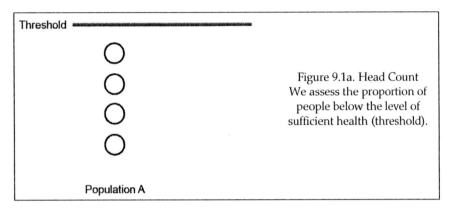

Figure 9.1a. Head Count
We assess the proportion of people below the level of sufficient health (threshold).

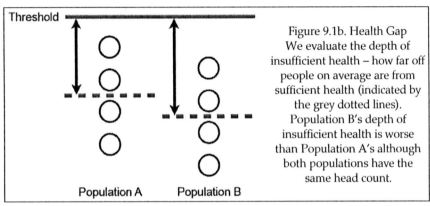

Figure 9.1b. Health Gap
We evaluate the depth of insufficient health – how far off people on average are from sufficient health (indicated by the grey dotted lines). Population B's depth of insufficient health is worse than Population A's although both populations have the same head count.

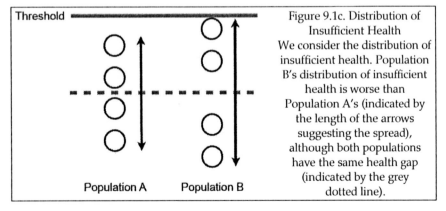

Figure 9.1c. Distribution of Insufficient Health
We consider the distribution of insufficient health. Population B's distribution of insufficient health is worse than Population A's (indicated by the length of the arrows suggesting the spread), although both populations have the same health gap (indicated by the grey dotted line).

Figures 9.1a, b and c Measuring insufficient health following the poverty literature.

For policy-making it is often useful to know not only how good or bad the degree of health inequity is but also which population sub-groups are affected by health inequity. Sub-group decomposition is one method to offer such information, and this is one attractive feature of the FGT measure.[7] In this analysis, I use sex, income and education as sub-group characteristics and examine the contribution of each sub-group (that is, male, female, each of the household income quintiles adjusted for the household size, and each of the four education sub-groups [less than high school; high school degree or equivalent; trades certification, vocational school or community college; university or college certificate]) to the total degree of health inequity based on a sufficiency view in the population.

Analysis
Separately for Canada and the US, I describe health inequity based on a sufficiency view using the FGT measure ($\alpha=0$, 1 and 2) for all ages and each of the three age groups (18–44, 45–64 and 65+ years). As a demonstration of the policy usefulness of the sub-group decomposition of the FGT measure, I then decompose health inequity measured by the FGT measure by sex, income and education for the middle age group (45–64 years). I select this age group because the empirical literature typically shows the greatest health inequity among the middle age. All models are weighted with the JCUSH survey weights. I use Stata 11 (StataCorp 2009; Jenkins 1999) for all analyses.

3.2 Results

The degree of health inequity based on a sufficiency view of health equity appears to be greater in the US than in Canada (Table 9.1). The sufficient level of health (set as the average health) is on the whole about the same in Canada and the United States (HUI=0.886 in Canada and 0.873 in the US for all age groups combined, the difference is less than the clinically significant cut-point of 0.030). The degree of health inequity measured by the FGT ($\alpha=2$) is greater in the US (0.047) than in Canada (0.038). In both countries, the sufficient levels of health between the three age groups are clinically significantly different, with a lower level for an older group. All three indicators of inequity – the head count (based on FGT [$\alpha=0$]), the health gap (based on FGT [$\alpha=1$]) and the distribution of insufficient health (based on FGT [$\alpha=2$])

– suggest that inequity is of most concern among the oldest age group (65+ years).

An examination of these three indicators reveals how inequity differs across the three age groups. In Canada, the average health gap is always worse in an older age group, while the proportion of those below sufficient health and health inequality among them are similar between the young adults (18–44 years) and the middle-aged adults (45–64 years). In the US, on the other hand, both the average health gap and health inequity among those below sufficient health are always worse in an older age group. The proportion of those below sufficient health is about the same across the young adults and the middle-aged adults. In both countries, a little over 30 per cent of people aged 65 or older are below sufficient health, and the average shortfall of health is about 0.300 in the HUI score (ten times more than the minimally clinically significant difference of 0.030). Considering the distribution of insufficient health, in this age group the degree of health inequity is greater in the US (0.088 in the FGT) than in Canada (0.076 in the FGT).

Sub-group decomposition analysis provides a profile of health inequity (Table 9.2). Among the middle-aged adults in both countries health inequity is worse among persons with lower socio-economic status (measured by income or education) by all three indicators (the FGT [$\alpha=0$, 1, and 2]). Health inequity among persons with lower socio-economic status is worse in the US than in Canada. In the US, close to 60 per cent of the lowest socio-economic status is below the sufficient level of health, the average shortfall of the HUI among those below sufficient level is 0.350 (more than ten times more than the minimally clinically significant difference of 0.030), and the degree of inequity measured by the FGT ($\alpha=2$) is 0.16. The contribution of the lowest income group to health inequity is 43 per cent, while that of the lowest education group is 23 per cent in the US. The smaller contribution indicated among the lowest education group than the lowest income group reflects the fact that the inequity contribution takes into account both the degree of inequity and the population share. The lowest education group exhibits the greatest inequity but has a small population share of 8 per cent. Health inequity profile by sex is less dramatic than that seen by socio-economic status. Inequity is slightly worse among women than men in both countries.

Table 9.1 Empirical application of a sufficiency view of health equity.

	N	Sufficient health (HUI)[a]	Head count[b] (Individuals below sufficient health, %)	Average health gap (HUI)[c]	Average health gap (% sufficient health)[d]	Degree of health inequity[e]
Canada						
All ages	2,891	0.886	25.57	0.239	6.91	0.038
18-44 years	1,439	0.910	26.80	0.193	5.69	0.030
45-64 years	918	0.882	26.69	0.218	6.61	0.031
65+ years	534	0.801	31.38	0.301	11.81	0.076
United States						
All ages	3,798	0.873	26.42	0.263	7.95	0.047
18-44 years	1,822	0.907	27.97	0.188	5.80	0.030
45-64 years	1,300	0.851	27.48	0.281	9.07	0.054
65+ years	671	0.786	32.41	0.319	13.14	0.088

[a] The average level of health in each category

[b] Based on FGT ($\alpha=0$)

[c] (Sufficient health) - (Average health among those below sufficient health)

[d] Based on FGT ($\alpha=1$)

[e] Based on FGT ($\alpha=2$)

Data source: 2002-3 Joint Canada-United States Survey of Health

Table 9.2 Subgroup decomposition analysis based on a sufficiency view of health equity.

	Population share (%)	Head count* (Individuals below sufficient health, %)	Average health gap		Degree of health inequity[d]	Contribution to total inequity (%)
			(HUI)[b]	(% sufficient healthy)[c]		
Canada						
Sex						
Female	48.53	30.34	0.214	7.35	0.034	52.96
Male	51.47	23.25	0.225	5.92	0.029	47.04
Total	100	26.69	0.218	6.61	0.031	100
Income						
Bottom quintile	14.64	50.00	0.308	17.45	0.100	46.50
2nd bottom quintile	17.46	33.20	0.217	8.17	0.041	22.97
Middle quintile	17.23	25.65	0.180	5.23	0.021	11.51
2nd top quintile	23.94	19.19	0.180	3.92	0.016	11.95
Top quintile	26.72	17.07	0.153	2.95	0.008	7.07
Total	100	26.69	0.218	6.61	0.031	100
Education						
Less than high school	19.23	36.07	0.265	10.83	0.058	35.54
High school degree or equivalent	27.16	29.43	0.217	7.25	0.033	28.85
Trades certification, vocational school, community college	22.42	27.59	0.213	6.65	0.032	22.91
University or college certificate	31.18	17.88	0.169	3.42	0.013	12.71
Total	100	26.69	0.218	6.61	0.031	100
United States						
Sex						
Female	50.45	28.97	0.272	9.26	0.057	53.51
Male	49.55	25.96	0.291	8.88	0.051	46.49
Total	100	27.48	0.281	9.07	0.054	100
Income						
Lowest	14.62	59.17	0.351	24.41	0.160	43.05
Lower middle	15.96	31.85	0.324	12.14	0.063	24.57
Middle	17.68	24.57	0.245	7.06	0.038	12.51
Upper middle	23.68	22.33	0.231	6.05	0.029	12.76
Highest	28.06	14.65	0.183	3.16	0.014	7.11
Total	100	27.48	0.281	9.07	0.054	100
Education						
Less than high school	7.53	56.06	0.352	23.16	0.156	21.72
High school degree or equivalent	34.12	33.45	0.285	11.21	0.068	43.10
Trades certification, vocational school, community college	15.35	28.67	0.302	10.18	0.062	17.62
University or college certificate	43.00	17.30	0.222	4.51	0.022	17.56
Total	100	27.48	0.281	9.07	0.054	100

Sufficient level of health (HUI) = 0.882 for Canada and 0.851 for the US
* Based on FGT (α=0)
[b](Sufficient health) - (Average health among those below sufficient health)
[c] Based on FGT (α=1)
[d] Based on FGT (α=2)
Data source: 2002-3 Joint Canada-United States Survey of Health

4. DISCUSSION

In this chapter I explored a sufficiency view of health equity as an alternative way to define health inequity by examining the *level* of health rather than the *causes* of health inequalities, as most of the work to date has done. Arguing for health sufficiency requires articulation of why and in what way we value health, and I found such articulation in understanding health as a capability. To apply a sufficiency view of health equity empirically, I used poverty analysis as a methodological foundation. Just as analyses of income inequality and poverty offer unique information in the sphere of income distribution, health sufficiency analyses can provide valuable information that is not obvious in analyses of the entire health distribution. This chapter planted seeds for this new approach, and I end this chapter by discussing below a few issues that arise in this exploration for further development of this view.

Compared to equity in access to or use of healthcare, where at least the concept of need, albeit with varying definitions, is accepted as central to define equity, equity in health outcomes is a muddled field. It is then reasonable to ask whether the field needs yet another definition or perspective of health inequity as I propose in this chapter. My response is twofold. First, my proposal of a sufficiency view of health equity is an attempt to capture a sentiment of health equity that has already been expressed in diverse literatures rather than suggesting something unexpected. Powers and Faden (2008) and Ruger (2010) are other examples of recent attempts to think about justice and health informed by the capabilities approach, and in his latest book, *Just Health* (Daniels 2008), Daniels also discusses similarities between the capabilities approach and his view of normal species functioning as a foundation for fair opportunity, extending John Rawls' theory of justice as fairness (1971). A merit of my exploration in this paper may then be how this growing sentiment of health equity can be further developed as a sufficiency view of health equity and how this view might serve as a basis for empirical application.

Second, a sufficiency view of health equity may offer at least a partial answer to the question of the moral significance of *univariate* health inequality. Around 2000, Christopher Murray, Emmanuela Gakidou and Julio Frenk, then at the World Health Organization, argued for the importance of examining and measuring health distribution only, regardless of its associations with other attributes, such as socio-economic status, race or ethnicity, or geographic location (Murray, Gakidou and Frenk 1999; World Health Organization 2000). In most epidemiological studies, health inequalities have traditionally been examined and measured as bivariate associations (for example, health–income, health–race, health–rurality, etc.). Their proposal, hence, caused a heated debate (Braveman, Krieger and Lynch 2000; Braveman, Starfield and Geiger 2001; Murray, Gakidou and Frenk 1999). Murray and his colleagues argued that health has intrinsic value and univariate health inequality is not just a variation but is an ethically significant variation, thus, inequitable. The opponents, a large majority of the empirical health inequity community, contended that what is morally significant in health inequality is the systematic associations between health and other attributes. Despite the heated debate, the moral significance of univariate health inequality has never been clearly articulated or penetrated in the health inequity field. A sufficiency view of health equity supported by the capabilities approach may offer one reason why we might consider that it is morally meaningful to examine health distribution only. It is because sufficient health is a capability, which our society perceives as an essential for every person to have to act as an equal citizen. The concept of sufficient health, thus, highlights the importance of health without negating the importance of correlations between health and other attributes.

The concept of a sufficiency view of health equity and its empirical application sketched out in this chapter suggest the definition of sufficient health and the use of a poverty measure as key issues for further development of this view. In this chapter I explored but did not defend particular solutions for the challenges of universality and infeasibility in defining sufficient health. Along with rigorous conceptual discussion regarding these challenges, it will be useful in future work to conduct sensitivity analyses examining how much difference the definition of sufficient health brings to empirical estimates of the degree of health inequity. Such sensitivity analyses will be particularly important when empirical application extends to global health data, including countries with vast differences in the technological advancement, available knowledge and resource constraint much more than those between Canada and the US. In addition, the use of the FGT measure as a measure of health inequity from a perspective of sufficient health requires further attention to effective communication. It is unfortunate that the degree of health inequity measured by the FGT measure ($\alpha=2$)

does not give natural, intuitive interpretation. While the lack of inter-pretability applies to many indices and a standard interpretation of an index usually develops among its users as its use increases, it will be valuable to develop effective communication strategies around the FGT measure. This will be particularly so when an empirical application of a sufficiency view goes beyond academic work and expands to policy-relevant work.

Notes

1. I am grateful for the comments and suggestions made by the participants of the International Studies Association (ISA) Health Inequalities and Global Justice Workshop in March 2011. I would also like to thank Ole Frithjof Norheim and Trygve Ottersen for their comments to an earlier version of this paper and Alyce Whipp for research and editorial assistance.
2. See Hausman in this volume for a discussion of the idea of responsibility underlying this approach.
3. From the defence of 'democratic equality' rather than compensation of undeserved bad luck as a fundamental starting point of the pursuit of egali-tarianism, Anderson supports capabilities as the appropriate focal point of justice. She, however, does not emphasise sufficiency as much as I do in this chapter.
4. The JCUSH Public Use Microdata File is publicly available from the US National Center for Health Statistics web page (http://www.cdc.gov/nchs/nhis/jcush.htm).
5. Excluded from the target population of the JCUSH were people in institu-tions, prisons, full-time Canadian or US Armed Forces personnel, or resi-dents of territories. The JCUSH was designed to provide reliable estimates at the national level for three age groups (18–44, 45–64 and 65+ years) by sex. Response rates were 65.5 per cent (Canada) and 50.2 per cent (US), and sample sizes were 3,505 (Canada) and 5,183 (US). The analysis presented in this chapter excludes observations with missing values.
6. Formally, the FGT measure (P_α) is defined as follows:

$$P_\alpha = \frac{1}{N} \sum_{i=1}^{n} \left(\frac{z-y_i}{z}\right)^\alpha$$

where N is the total population, n is the number of people below the suf-ficient level of health, $y=(y_1, y_2, ..., y_N)$ is a vector of health in increasing order, z is the sufficient level of health, and $z-y_i$ is the health shortfall of the ith individual. α is a measure of the sensitivity to the health gap and takes values equal to or greater than zero. A larger α indicates a greater weight assigned to sicker individuals below the sufficient health. For all $\alpha = 0$, 1, or and 2, the FGT measure takes values between 0 and 1. For the FGT ($\alpha=0$), 0 means no one is below the sufficient health while 1 means everyone is below the sufficient health. For the FGT ($\alpha=1$), 0 suggests no shortfall at all, and 1 suggests 100 per cent shortfall. A smaller value of the FGT measure ($\alpha=2$) suggests a greater achievement of health equity based on a sufficiency view although, unlike $\alpha=0$ (measuring the proportion of people with insufficient health) and $\alpha=1$ (measuring the average shortfall), it does not provide intuitive interpretation.

7. Suppose data contain sub-groups j = 1, 2, …, m. The FGT measure (P_α) can be decomposed by sub-group population as follows:

$$P_\alpha = \sum_{j=1}^{m} \frac{N_j}{N} \cdot P_\alpha^j$$

where Nj is the total population of sub-group j, is the FGT measure for the sub-group j.

Chapter 10

RATING EFFORTS TO EXTEND ACCESS ON ESSENTIAL MEDICINES: INCREASING GLOBAL HEALTH IMPACT[1]

Nicole Hassoun

INTRODUCTION

Global inequality impacts global health. The rich can, but the poor cannot, access many of the existing medicines they need. About a third of all deaths, 18 million a year or 50,000 every day, are poverty-related (World Health Organization 2004). There is also a large mismatch between pharmaceutical research and development (R&D) spending and the global burden of disease (GBD) (Lichtenberg 2005: 663–90; Culp and Hassoun forthcoming). Pharmaceutical companies have very little incentive to do new R&D on drugs for the poor (who lack the money to buy them). What should we do to address the consequences of inequality for global health?

One option is to restructure the incentives pharmaceutical companies face so that they can extend access on essential medicines to the poor. Many have argued that this is morally required (Hollis and Pogge 2008: Flory and Kitcher 2004: 36–65). To date, however, very few philosophers have advanced concrete proposals for doing so.[2] Though, many have criticised Thomas Pogge's proposal for a Health Impact Fund that would provide prizes for companies producing new drugs in proportion to their impact on global health (Pogge 2008a). That more philosophical work has not been done on this topic is unfortunate. To begin to fill this lacuna, this chapter considers the case for a new alternative: rating companies' efforts to extend access on essential medicines on the basis of the disease burden their innovations might alleviate, their effectiveness, and how many people have access to them.

As I argue elsewhere, a good rating system will incentivise companies to promote global health (Hassoun forthcoming (a); Hassoun forthcoming (b)). Highly rated companies might, for instance, be given a Global Health Impact (GHI) label to use on all of their – especially over-the-counter – products. This label might be similar to 'Fair Trade', '(Product) RED', 'USDA Organic' or 'Ethos' labels. Highly rated companies might use the GHI label to garner a larger share of the market, as people prefer goods from 'ethically' labelled companies (Reynolds 2002). If Pfizer, for example, was highly rated, it could use the label on all of its products, including Advil. If even a small percentage of consumers would prefer products from highly rated companies, the incentive to use the GHI label for analgesics alone could be significant in this approximately US$2 billion a year market (Reynolds 2002). Furthermore, pharmaceutical companies make many products besides drugs – from diet drinks and lotion, to pet vitamins and mouth wash. So, they could use the GHI label on these products too.

Even if a labelling campaign is not a good idea, a GHI rating system should be of intrinsic interest and would open the door to other ways of incentivising innovation. Pharmaceutical companies and researchers might use it to gauge R&D efforts. Socially responsible investment organisations could include GHI companies in their portfolios. One can also imagine boycotts of poorly rated companies, lobbying of insurance companies to include GHI products in their formularies, and so forth. Finally, because pharmaceutical companies rely on university R&D, universities might make it a condition of the sale of their licences that companies agree to abide by GHI standards. If such a GHI Licensing Campaign was only as successful as United Students Against Sweatshops has been so far in convincing campuses to change their licensing practices, this proposal will create US$840 million worth of incentive for pharmaceutical companies to become certified every year (Reynolds 2002: 71; Hassoun forthcoming (a)). That is about the cost of developing a new drug on the highest estimates.[3] This much money might greatly increase the rate of new drugs development for neglected diseases (Trouiller et al. 2002: 945–51). This proposal will not solve every health problem but, if successful, it will have a significant impact on some of them (Broome 2005).[4]

This paper argues that it is possible to design a good rating system – one that rewards highly rated companies for doing things that actually promote global health. It also suggests that practical work on promoting global health can yield interesting philosophical questions and conclusions by highlighting some of the normative choices that it is important to address in developing a rating system.

RATING SYSTEM DESIGN

To rate companies on the basis of some of their products' impact it is first necessary to decide exactly which drugs, diseases, and population groups to focus on. In previous work, I suggested looking at the US Food and Drug Administration approved 'orphan' drugs. (Orphan drugs are, roughly, drugs that are not expected to have large markets in the US) (FDA 2008). I no longer believe this is the best way to proceed. Too many things that are important for global health are absent from the list. The only malaria drugs on the orphan drug list, for instance, are Mefloquine (Larium), Quinine Sulfate and Halofantrine (BIO Ventures for Global Health 2011).[5] There are twenty-three (often combination) treatments for (primarily, p. falciparum or p. vivax) malaria that the World Health Organization (WHO) found worth examining for resistance and efficacy (WHO 2010). It is probably better just to consider some of the drugs for diseases that have a large impact on the poor – neglected tropical diseases, malaria, HIV, tuberculosis and so forth. Though, which diseases have the largest impact on the poor depends, in part, on what counts as a disease (or how the diseases are grouped). In WHO calculations, for instance, diarrhoeal diseases (rotavirus, cholera, dysentery, etc.) are grouped and, so, have a much bigger impact in terms of mortality (and other measures of disease burden) than they would each have alone. Similarly, the impact of childhood diseases looks significant because they are grouped together, but most do not have a large impact on their own. Fortunately, there may be room for pragmatic considerations to enter into choosing some sub-set of diseases to focus on in developing a rating system.

Supposing it is possible to settle on a list of diseases by appeal to pragmatic considerations, hard questions remain about which drugs and population groups to focus on. A reasonable first approximation might be to look at the impact of first-line drugs for those diseases in all the countries where the disease is prevalent (by comparing existing first-line drugs to the next best available drug). This is a reasonable place to start, even though there are different ways of defining the poorest countries, and sometimes drugs that do not address the diseases prevalent in these countries will have a large impact on global health. There is good evidence that companies often neglect the diseases prevalent in these countries (Lichtenberg 2005: 663–90; Culp and

Hassoun forthcoming). So, there is reason for those interested in promoting global health to encourage companies to focus on addressing this oversight.

One might object to limiting the study to any sub-set of drugs or diseases, especially as this will increase global inequality in some respects. Even inequality among the poor may rise if not every disease that afflicts poor people is on the list. More generally, one might worry about creating a rating system for only some of the things companies are doing (extending access on essential medicines to the poor as opposed to improving health infrastructure or whatnot). For a partial rating system will give companies an incentive to divert funds to meeting only some needs.

This may not, however, pose an ethical problem. It may be permissible for individual researchers and non-governmental organisations (NGOs) working on a label to do what they can to encourage companies to extend access on some drugs for malaria or neglected tropical diseases. This may just provide reason for others to encourage companies to extend access on other medicines or to make appropriate health-related infrastructure investments or whatnot. After all, the money that companies put into extending access on some medicines need not undermine their other attempts to help the poor. The GHI labelling proposal advanced here is not a complete solution to the problems the poor face in meeting their basic health needs. Still, it may *help* the poor meet these needs.

Moreover, once there is some rating system in place, it may be possible to elicit more information as a condition of rating companies. Some information (for example, about drug prices) is sensitive, but the proposal gives companies an incentive to release it.

Supposing we can arrive at a select list of diseases and focus drugs, some of the standard tools for effectiveness analysis may allow us to evaluate companies on that basis. The proposed methodology is, roughly, this. First, consider the burden of disease alleviated by each drug in the relevant countries, for example in disability adjusted life-years (DALYs). The burden of disease equivalent dosages will alleviate can be calculated using a proxy for access like price, the disease burden information in the WHO's burden of disease (GBD) study, and drug efficacy estimates modelled from efficacy data collected from WHO reports, clinical trials and meta-analyses of such data (the necessary modelling is sketched in the next section). Consider an illustrative example of how this information might be used. Suppose, for simplicity's sake, that everyone has access to all of the drugs evaluated.[6] Suppose disease burden is calculated in DALYs and 34 million DALYs are lost to plasmodium falciparum malaria. Suppose Quinine is effective in about 9 per cent of cases while Mefloquine is effective in about 5 per cent of cases. If the next best alternative to each of these drugs averted 1 million DALYs, at the margin Quinine and Mefloquine might avert about 2.1 and 0.7 million DALYs respectively. The next step is to rate companies on the basis of their inventions' (marginal potential) impact. Suppose Pfizer has two drugs that, at the margin, avert the loss of 2.1 and 0.7 million DALYs respectively. Suppose Bayer has one drug that, at the margin, averts the loss of 3 million DALYs. Bayer may be ranked above Pfizer. The marginal impact of Bayer's drug is 3 million DALYs averted, while Pfizer's drugs' marginal impact is 2.8 million DALYs averted. If innovations are evaluated in this way, this rating system will give companies an incentive to produce more effective drugs that address the largest global health problems.

Michael Selgelid might object to looking at drugs' *marginal* impact. Some drugs have a greater impact in combination than alone. Looking at marginal impact is to suppose one particular way of splitting the credit between companies' interventions but it is not clearly the best way. To illustrate the problem, suppose that we decide to measure disease burden in DALYs. Suppose one company's drug averts 2 million DALYs on its own. Then, suppose another company creates a drug that would alleviate 1 million DALYs on its own, but together with the first company's drug helps avert 20 million DALYs. Should the new intervention receive credit for averting 18 million DALYs and the original intervention receive credit for averting 2 million DALYs? Should the 18 million marginal gain be split between the interventions? Should the new company receive all 20 million in credit?

It may be morally acceptable to attribute credit in many ways, but it is clear how the question should be answered in this context. What matters is maximising the incentive for companies to ameliorate the GBD. If the recommended treatment becomes a combination of two drugs, one might initially think the company producing the new drug should get all the credit for the marginal impact of its creation (18 million DALYs averted). If another company comes along and offers a better drug to be used in combination with the original drug – that, say, saves 21 million DALYs – that company would then receive 1 million DALYs' worth of credit and the other company would receive none.

Selgelid worries that this will give companies an incentive not to put their part of a combination forward (or to withdraw it from the market) until other companies put their part of the combination forward, but I am not sure this will pose a problem for the rating system. Companies that make drugs that might be used in combination have reason to negotiate with each other to bring the new interventions forward as soon as possible. The company that expects to make the most from delay will, in theory, just pay the other company, or companies, to be the last one to release the intervention.[7] If, however, things do not work out so well in practice, the rating might be amended to apportion credit differently. It is also possible to refrain from crediting companies that are charged with delaying the entry of their drugs onto the market (or withdrawing their drugs from the market) when this does not benefit, or instead harms, the poor (Selgelid 2008).

If this issue can be resolved, the main challenge for estimating existing products' impact is to develop good proxies for burden, effectiveness and access. A good proxy is one that both tracks the variable of interest and, if manipulated by companies, would yield good results for the poor. Moreover, it must be possible for companies to affect the proxy. One of the things that makes choosing good proxies difficult is that burden, effectiveness and access are connected. Given that not everyone can access every drug, for instance, it is not clear how we can tell how effective the drug is for those who do secure it. Nevertheless, subsequent sections will consider just a few of the issues that arise in choosing good proxies for burden, effectiveness and access independently.

MEASURING BURDEN

One of the main constraints in determining the disease burden any particular intervention might alleviate (as well as access to that intervention and its effectiveness) is data at the global level. Perhaps the best source for burden of disease information is the Institute for Health Metric and Evaluation's GBD study (now supported by the WHO and the Gates Foundation), although even this study lacks information on many diseases. Again, it may be acceptable to narrow the rating system's focus for pragmatic reasons – researchers might consider only those diseases that have a large impact in developing countries that appear on the GBD list. For there is little global data using other measures of disease burden like quality adjusted life-years (QUALYs) and the GBD study is one of the best and most comprehensive sources of global burden of disease information available.

Even if we limit our attention to deciding between the available measures of disease burden for which global health data is available through the GBD study, a few questions remain. We must first decide, for instance, whether to use DALYs or the years of life lost (YLL) to a disease. Very roughly, DALYs are YLL to disease plus years lost to disability (YLD) (Murray 1996). The YLL is, roughly, a standard life expectation (for women and men) minus the age at death.[8] The most common (incidence) measure of YLD is roughly disease duration times incidence and disability weight.

If we must choose between using DALYs or (different estimates of) YLL to a disease, an advantage of using DALYs is that they include some information about the burden of disability due to disease. Some diseases are terrible but do not kill their victims. If the disease burden was only measured in YLL, companies would receive no credit for curing or ameliorating these diseases.

Consider how DALYs are constructed. The original disability weights in the GBD study were based on healthcare providers' judgements about how bad different disabilities are compared with one another and mortality rates at the population level. Experts were asked questions like: 'If you had to choose between providing a medication that would extend the life of 1,000 healthy people by one year or 2,000 blind people by one year, which would you do?' (Murray and Acharya 1997: 703–30; Murray, Salomon and Mathers 2002).[9] These judgements were made after discussion with other healthcare providers at an international conference. The experts were asked to give consistent preference rankings. The GBD study's justification for constructing DALYs in this way appealed to the axiom that the burden of disease for similar health outcomes should be identical – that is, that the only non-health factors that are relevant are age and sex. The methodology continues to evolve.

There are some philosophical issues with the construction of DALYs that are worth noting (King and Bertino 2008: 209).[10] The first is that it is not at all clear whose preferences are the most reliable guides to the actual burden of death and disability.[11] Those who are sick or disabled (henceforth, simply *disabled*) often believe that their disabilities are not as bad as others believe them to be. They often have more knowledge about the relevant possibilities (phenomenological as well as factual) but, some argue, their opinions may be distorted by the fact that they have adapted to their poor condition (Murray and Acharya 1997: 703–30; Murray, Salomon and Mathers 2002). It really matters whose opinions are used in the current context (though different measures for the size of the burden of disease and what we should do about it may be necessary). If disabilities get less weight in DALY estimates then, on the proposed rating system, companies will get more credit for saving the lives of disabled people but less credit for alleviating their disability. This is because, in effect, disabled peoples' lives are discounted by the weight of their disability in the DALY calculations. Suppose for instance that, given that deaf people assign deafness a lower disability weight than non-deaf people, a company that helps a deaf person hear will avert 10 rather than 20 DALYs. Suppose another company saves the life of that deaf person but does not cure his or her deafness, and saving the life of an (otherwise similar) non-deaf person would be worth 30 DALYs. Once we consider the fact that some DALYs would still be lost to deafness, the second company will get 20 DALYs' worth of credit for saving the deaf person's life if we use the deaf people's evaluation (30–10). The second company will only get 10 DALYs' worth of credit for saving the deaf person's life on the non-deaf people's evaluation (30–20). Even if the preferences of the disabled *should* ultimately get priority, however, there are no alternative weights provided (for example, by disabled people) with which we might try to arrive at a better estimate of DALYs lost to different diseases.

Still, if DALYs are selected, it is possible to choose between two ways of calculating them (incidence and prevalence measures), whether to discount them and whether to use age-weighted DALYs. Discounting (by 3 per cent in the GBD study) gives less weight to the benefit of interventions' impacts in the future, while the age-weighting in the GBD study gives more credit to interventions that benefit those in early adulthood as opposed to children or the elderly. Consider each of these issues in turn.

In trying to measure the DALYs lost to a disease in a given year, incidence and prevalence DALYs deal in different ways with the burden of disabilities. Prevalence DALYs include the disability people experience in that year as a result of their disease (whenever these people acquired the disease). Incidence DALYs include a projection of the present and future disability attributable to disease *acquired* in the relevant year (Murray and Acharya 1997: 703–30; Murray, Salomon and Mathers 2002).[12] An example will help illustrate the difference.[13] Suppose that there are two 40-year-old men and we want to know the DALYs lost in 2004 and each of the next forty years in which they are expected to live.

Man 1 acquires a disease in 2004 that kills him.

Man 2 acquires a disease in 2004 that moderately disables him.

Suppose the weight associated with moderate disability is .25. The weight associated with death is 1 for each year a person would otherwise be expected to be alive. Prevalence DALYs suggest that 40 years of life are lost, in 2004, to the disease that afflicts Man 1. Prevalence DALYs suggest that the equivalent of .25 years are lost, in 2004, to the disability that results from the disease that afflicts Man 2. In 2005 and so forth, only the equivalent of .25 years would be lost to the disease that afflicts Man 2 (because no new health problems arise in those years and Man 2's disease remains prevalent in each of those years). Incidence DALYs suggest that forty years of life are lost, in 2004, to the disease that afflicts Man 1. Incidence DALYs suggest that the equivalent of 10 years are lost, in 2004, due to disability from the disease that afflicts Man 2 (.25*40). In 2005 and so forth, no DALYs are lost. Prevalence DALYs consider the total impact of death in a given year but consider the disability experienced in that year that may have been acquired much earlier. Incidence DALYs consider the total impact of death and disability that happens in a given year.

The difference between using incidence and prevalence DALYs might not be important if we do not discount DALYs (Murray and Acharya 1997: 703–30; Murray, Salomon and Mathers 2002).[14] With discounting, however, this difference is significant. These measures will not only yield different estimates of disease burden but will give different weight to some diseases over others. Though, on both measures the impact of interventions in the future will be less (that is just the effect of discounting). Consider an example from Drew Schroeder's important paper 'Prevalence, Incidence, and Hybrid Approaches to Calculating DALYs'. Suppose there are two diseases. The first one afflicts 100 people a year and causes a serious disability with a disability weight of .5. The resulting disability lasts for one year. The second disease afflicts two people per year and also causes a serious disability with a disability weight of .5 but the resulting disability lasts for 50 years. Suppose that, since the second disease has been around long enough, 100 people have it at any point in time. At any given time, both diseases cause 50 DALYs to be lost if we do not discount whether we use incidence or prevalence DALYs (.5*100). If we use discounted prevalence DALYs, both diseases will still be judged equally burdensome. If we use discounted incidence DALYs, however, the first disease will look almost twice as bad as the second (at standard discount rates). It is hard to see why the first disease should be counted as worse than the second in terms of the global disease burden (once the second has been around long enough). The second yields just as much disability in every year. So, if we discount DALYs, there is some reason to use a prevalence measure.[15]

But, should we discount? One rationale for discounting is to track individuals' preferences. People may prefer to give more weight to earlier rather than later health benefits (Murray and Acharya 1997: 703–30; Murray, Salomon and Mathers 2002). Fortunately, we need not consider whether this argument is sustainable, or other philosophical arguments for or against discounting the future, to conclude that there is some reason to discount.[16] In the current context, uncertainty about what health interventions will be developed in the future provides reason to discount. Drug resistance and new drug development tend to make existing interventions obsolete. Any projected credit companies receive should be discounted for the chance that their interventions will alleviate less health burden into the future. This might, more precisely, be reason to discount estimates of drug effectiveness. However, discounting DALYs will achieve the same result. The proposed rating system is Burden*Effectiveness*Access and discounting enters into the equation multiplicatively. Although much more reflection on this topic is necessary, there is at least one reason to discount.[17]

Finally, consider age-weighting. In the GBD study, more weight is given to the disease burden for adults than for children or the elderly. This is because, in some studies, people give preference to years of life lived as a young adult (though the evidence here is quite mixed) (Murray and Acharya 1997: 703–30; Murray, Salomon and Mathers 2002). One objection to age-weighting is that it treats some lives as more valuable than others (Anand and Hanson 1997: 685–702; Murray and Acharya 1997: 703–30; Murray, Salomon and Mathers 2002). The fact that the authors assume that all individuals potentially live through every life stage does not allay this worry. When YLD are calculated, the effects of disease on those who die young receive less weight. Moreover, insofar as the aim is to give companies an incentive to ameliorate disease in the future, this measure will encourage them to focus on helping young adults. If they do so, those who die young will not benefit as much as they would if companies focused equally on the needs of children. If we should treat all people equally, perhaps we should not incentivise companies to address diseases that impact young adults in particular. One possible response to this objection is that the population structure in developing countries is skewed towards younger populations, so if the age-weighting better approximates the population structure in these countries, age-weighting may be appropriate as a way of achieving equal treatment across age groups (Lopez et al. 2006). Unfortunately, there is little reason to think that age-weighting will get the population structure right (even for the average disease in the study), as there are usually many children in developing countries. To treat all people equally, it makes more sense to apply age-weights that reflect the population age structure in each country using population life tables for these countries (for example, to weight age groups by their proportion in each country's population) (United Nations 1986).[18]

One might object that the preceding argument required a commitment to rewarding companies for helping all people equally. If doing so does not give them an incentive to reduce the GBD as much as possible, perhaps that commitment is unsustainable in this context.

Unless there is reason to believe that age-weighted DALYs are more accurate than unweighted DALYs in measuring the burden of disease, however, this objection fails. There is no reason to think we must choose between using a more accurate measure of disease burden and giving companies an incentive to help all people equally (Lopez et al. 2006).[19]

Although much more consideration is warranted, philosophical reflection can help select the best available measure of disease burden for constructing a good rating system (Arnesen and Nord 1999: 1423–5). Such inquiry might suggest using discounted prevalence DALYs (perhaps weighted by population life tables) in countries where the intervention being evaluated is a first-line therapy. At least, the above arguments provide some reason to accept this conclusion. The next section will suppose that that measure is selected and consider how to measure effectiveness and access to get an estimate of companies' drugs' (marginal potential) impact on the GBD.

MEASURING EFFECTIVENESS

Consider how to estimate drug effectiveness. The obvious proxy is efficacy in clinical trials. Clinical trial data may not reflect real-world drug efficacy. People may be more likely to adhere to treatment regimes in trials, they may receive additional medical care or other benefits, and even the quality of the medicines may be different. Unfortunately, there is currently no easily accessible, comparable, global efficacy information outside of clinical trial results. So although there may be reason to try to get more accurate estimates in the future, clinical trial results may provide a good starting point.

Some meta-analyses of efficacy data are available for some diseases but it is possible to supplement these studies with additional country-level data. Consider, for instance, some of the efficacy data on some malaria drugs' impact. This is available from the WHO's Global Report on Antimalarial Drug Efficacy and Drug Resistance 2000–10. It is also possible to find efficacy information from clinical trials conducted in many countries. Below is a graph with both the country/regional efficacy data and the WHO's Global Report on Antimalarial Drug Efficacy and Drug Resistance 2000–10 data for Chloroquine (WHO 2011).

The next step is to develop the methodology for combining this data and estimating missing data. The global efficacy estimates used in the general explanation of how to design a rating system were simple averages of regional estimates, but it is better to calculate a closer approximation (Hay et al. 2009). Drug effectiveness depends on many things related to different geographic locations (in some climates, for instance, the disease is more or less prevalent and stable and this affects transmission rates and affected individuals' parasite loads, which affects drug efficacy).[20] Very roughly, one possible way of trying to combine the data is by categorising each geographical area using estimates of transmission potential derived from vector ecology data (the ME index available from The Earth Institute at Columbia University) and other variables of relevance to drug efficacy for which it is possible to acquire global data.[21] This will provide the basis for developing a causal model (using regression analysis), in collaboration with experts in biostatistics, with which to impute efficacy estimates to different geographical

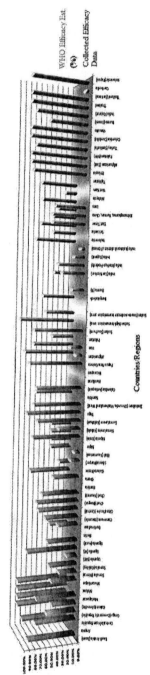

Figure 10.1 WHO and collected data on chloroquine efficacy by country/region.

regions using the collected efficacy data.[22] Other relevant information includes the size and quality of the study, the year in which it was conducted, the treatment group and what the drug at issue was compared with (if anything) in the study. Resulting efficacy estimates for all geographical regions will be combined to yield a global efficacy estimate. For the potential uses of the rating system described in the introduction, the results must be precise enough that, once drugs' impacts are aggregated, they issue a consistent ordinal ranking of companies. The dis-aggregated data might also be useful for guiding targeting interventions.[23]

MEASURING ACCESS

The obvious proxy for access is price, though price is certainly not the only barrier to access and there are different barriers in different circumstances. Affordability, availability, accessibility, accommodation and acceptability all affect access (Penchansky and Thomas 1981: 127–40). So, one might think a good proxy should be disease- or drug-specific. In some cases, price may be the biggest barrier to access, and so measuring price alone might be sufficient. In other cases, health infrastructure might be the biggest problem and it may be possible to reward companies for collaborating with partners in the developing world who have the ability to deliver their drugs to those in need. The problem with disease-specific proxies is that they may not be comparable between cases. How does a price of $3.50 per Chloroquine pill compare with providing 3,000 people with measles vaccine for free through a drug donation programme? Although it might, in principle, be possible to compare the impact of things like health infrastructure improvements and new public–private partnerships in terms of DALYs saved, doing so would be incredibly difficult. It may be hard even to measure the impact of some of the things companies are doing to improve access. It may be hard to tell, for instance, how much credit a company should get for giving drugs at a small cost to another company with the ability to distribute (and profit from) distributing their medicine to the poor. So, it might be better to limit the scope of the project by focusing only on certain barriers to access, at least initially.

Even if price is the selected proxy for access, it may take some work just to estimate global drug prices. Companies are reluctant to provide this information. In part this is because prices vary significantly in

Country	Comparator	Study Area	Sample Size	Age & Sex	Year	Other	Efficacy
Chad	SP, AQ	urban centres Bongor & Kourma, southern Chad	301/318 eligible for analysis	6-59 months	2006	more efficacious treatment needed; artesunate + AQ potential 1st-line treatment	76.3%
W Uganda	SP, SP + CQ	Kamwezi health centre and Kyogo sub-dispensary in Kamwezi sub-county in Kabale district, western Uganda	141	> 6 months most over 5 years	October of 2001	CQ still effective, but combo therapy SP + CQ recommended to delay SP resistance	92.5%
Uganda (rural)	SP, SP + CQ	Kaberamaido District, NE Uganda	104/117 had complete follow-up	median age 15 months	Third quarter of 2001	combo therapy most effective; increased CQ efficacy with age = developing some immunity	55.0%
Congo (Democratic Republic)	SP	Seven sites: Kinshasa, Mikalayi, Kapolowe, Vanga, Kimpese, Kisangani, Bukavu	499 ACR	children < 5 yrs	May 2000-Nov 2001	CQ no longer effective in Congo - SP new 1st line treatment	54.6%
Gabon	AQ	Libreville	63	children	Sept 1997-Jan 1998	AQ generally more effective than CQ	45.0%
Mali	SP	Koumantou	224	children	2003-2004	based combo therapy recommended	9.5%
Mozambique	AQ + SP, artesunate + SP, AQ + artesunate	Manhica district	Two studies 80/50	6-59 months	Feb-June 2001/2002	AQ more effective than SP than CQ, combo therapy 100% clinical efficacy	47.1%

Figure 10.2 Sample of initial collected efficacy data for chloroquine.[24]

different contexts and companies do not want their customers and competitors to access this information. Fortunately, there are a couple of ways around this problem. It might be possible to work with non-governmental and governmental organisations focusing on health, like the World Health Organization, Médecins Sans Frontières or health ministries, to secure a broad range of pricing information. The global fund provides information on the prices for many medications, as do many health ministries.[25] One nice thing about some country-level regulatory bodies – for example, in Colombia, Canada and Brazil – is that they have done reference-based pricing. That means that their prices are set on the basis of other companies' prices. So, relying on their prices as a proxy provides some information about prices in countries in their region.

If decent price data is available, it may be important to take into account how often the treatment must be administered over the course of the average (for example, sick) individual's life. A drug that is given at birth and prevents all future infection may, in effect, cost less than one that has to be given yearly. Perhaps a reasonable estimate of access would be $1/($price per dose$^*c^*$# of times it must be given$)$. The scaling term, c, may just be necessary to ensure that lower prices (less than a dollar per dose) continue to increase (rather than decrease) impact. Though, perhaps a scaling term should also modulate the impact of price in the rating system to capture its importance compared with disease burden and efficacy in reducing the GBD.[26]

If necessary, it is possible to work without information about access and focus on the question: How much good would companies' drugs do if everyone had them? This is still valuable information. It provides a measure of drug quality in light of disease burden. It would be a significant improvement over the status quo if companies focused on producing high-quality drugs that could alleviate large burdens. There is even an argument that that is all companies are responsible for doing. Others, for example governments or non-governmental organisations, should help fill the breach and provide those drugs to people who need them. Although I believe that this argument is, ultimately, mistaken – it would be best if companies provided drugs that actually alleviate disease burden – potentially useful drugs are still important.[27] Others may help provide them to people in need and, eventually, after the drugs come off patent and technology progresses, they may benefit poor people (in future generations).[28]

Note, however, that whether or not access is included, the design of a rating system poses difficult questions about relative concern for people in present and future generations. There may be a trade-off between giving credit for widely available and more effective drugs. Alternatively, given resistance rates and changes in disease prevalence and impact, we might have to decide how to specify rewards for drugs that we expect to alleviate larger burdens in the future than in the present. One way of starting to do so is to develop a model of expected present and future drug impact and then consider the realm of possible ethical decisions very carefully.

CONCLUSION

This paper has outlined a rating system for pharmaceutical companies' efforts to extend access on essential medicines to the poor. In doing so, it argued that practical work on promoting global health can yield interesting new philosophical questions and conclusions. For, what normative questions arise, and what answers are appropriate, depends significantly on what one is trying to achieve. More importantly, however, such a rating system might provide the basis for reducing inequality in global health and saving millions of lives.

Notes

1. I owe thanks to Yukiko Asada, Thomas Pogge, Peter Spirtes, Drew Schroeder, Darrel Moellendorf, Alex London, Barbara Buckinx, Bruce Lee, Thom Sergerson and Jocelyn Mackie for extremely helpful discussion, as well as those who commented on the initial proposal for work forthcoming in *Globalization and Justice: Shrinking Distance, Expanding Obligations* with Cambridge University Press and *Developing World Bioethics*. I am very thankful to the editors of these works for allowing me to draw on that material here. Moreover, I would like to thank the audience at the Center for Advanced Studies in Frankfurt as well as to the Center Justitia Amplificata, the Falk and Bekman Foundations, and Academics Stand Against Poverty for supporting my research on this project. A portion of the piece is adapted from an earlier chapter of mine, 'Pharmaceutical Justice', published in *The Encyclopedia of Global Justice*, ed. Deen K. Chatterjee (Springer 2011).
2. The main exception is Hollis and Pogge, *The Health Impact Fund, Making New Medicines Accessible for All: A Report of Incentives for Global Health*.

Though, there are many innovative proposals in the public policy literature.

3. This estimate assumes that 30 per cent of the drugs these companies rely on are coming from universities and is in line with other authors' estimates. Marcia Angell reports, for instance, that 'In 2002, for example, Pfizer licensed in 30 per cent of its drugs, and Merck 35 per cent (Angell 2004).'

4. This proposal is feasible and has some advantages over the main competitors. It can, in any case, be used in conjunction with all of the alternatives.

5. Though, with the recent introduction of priority review vouchers, this may change.

6. It may also be necessary to consider the problems associated with medicines in estimating their net benefits.

7. In the US, combination therapies have to be tested and FDA-approved together.

8. There are important philosophical questions about whether this is justified. That said, the difference they postulate is small and there is no easily available information on disease burden without this population bias.

9. There are many methods for eliciting preferences, including persontradeoff, time-tradeoff and standard gamble. The methods used continue to evolve.

10. A serious practical problem is about how the study deals with comorbidities. There are also reasons to believe the GBD study greatly under-estimates the impact of many diseases on the poor. Poor countries often lack good data and the authors are conservative in estimating impact from poor data. This may not be a problem for the purposes of the model, however, if there is little data for *all* of the diseases it includes.

11. For philosophical reflection on the role of preferences in DALYs more generally, see Hausman (2006).

12. Seasonal variation in prevalence is often taken into account in estimating annual prevalence.

13. For a similar example and a very nice introduction to the distinction and its significance, see Schroeder (2011).

14. Though, the method may have a big impact in some cases. See Hyder and Morrow 1999: 43–5.

15. Some think it is conceptually incoherent to take different (incidence and prevalence) perspectives on death and disability as prevalence DALYs do, though I am not sure why this is a problem.

16. For an interesting philosophical argument against discounting, see Broome 2005: 399–413.

17. It may not be reasonable to discount the impact of all interventions at the same rate.

18. More recent data is available from the WHO which presents life tables as a link on the country pages in their *Global Health Observatory*, available at http://www.who.int/countries/en/

19. Moreover, some ways of reducing disease burden may be better than others because, for instance, they help all people equally. There may be reason to credit companies more for reducing the burden in a better way.

20. Disease transmission in the area may be stable or unstable (sensitive or insensitive to natural and man-made perturbations), and the disease can be holo-, hyper-, meso- or hypo-endemic. This can impact which population sub-groups acquire the disease, how severe it is, and so forth (Hay, Smith and Snow 2008: 369–78).

21. Vector ecology is plausibly exogenous to drug efficacy.

22. It is, obviously, necessary to include an error term to account for those variables which are important but on which there is no global data and to do the requisite econometric analysis.

23. So far this paper has considered how to estimate drug impact only in a single year, but it may be possible to estimate effectiveness over longer periods of time. Since different drugs are effective for different lengths of time and different disease stages, information about the required treatment regime might be incorporated into an estimate of access. Though, this will raise a host of philosophical questions about, for instance, the separability of times in valuing health states, the importance of impacts on present and future generations, and so forth. See Broome 2002; Brock 2002; Griffin 2002.

24. The abbreviation SP is Sulfadoxine-Pyrimethamine, C is Chloroquine, Q is Quinine, and A is Amodiaquine. ACR indicates that the participants achieved adequate clinical results.

25. See, for instance, the Global Fund's information on regional prices (The Global Fund 2010). Brazil's ministry of health (Ministerio de Salud) publishes a list of prices for popular medicines: (Brasil Ministerio de Salud 2011). Also see South African Department of Health's *Database of Medicine Prices* (South African Department of Health 2011).

26. Information on average age of onset used in calculating the GBD and, in conjunction with life tables and treatment regimes, may be useful in estimating how often the treatments must be administered in the population.

27. One reason it may not be a good idea to focus on price is if third parties, like the global fund, bear the burden of lower prices.

28. This is not certain.

Part 4

Borders and Health

Chapter 11

JUSTICE AND HEALTH INEQUALITIES IN HUMANITARIAN CRISES: STRUCTURED HEALTH VULNERABILITIES AND NATURAL DISASTERS[1]

Ryoa Chung and Matthew R. Hunt

INTRODUCTION

The ways that individuals and communities are affected by humanitarian crises are the result of a matrix of determinants including various forms of inequality (O'Keefe 1976). These features create gradients of vulnerability – unequal susceptibility for incurring additional wrongs (Hurst 2008) – both within and between populations. Pre-existing inequalities are exacerbated in the context of catastrophes; disasters do not affect people equally and those that are already marginalised or disadvantaged (because of gender, ethnic, religious or socio-economic divides), in poor health or in precarious social situations, are likely to experience greater deprivation and harm. That vulnerability to catastrophe is determined by social, cultural and economic factors, and that catastrophes widen existing inequalities, is clear. It is less clear how these understandings should map on to programming and prioritisation for humanitarian medical assistance, and how questions of justice should be addressed by non-governmental organisations (NGOs) involved in the medical response to natural disasters in low resource settings.

In this paper, we argue that health vulnerabilities that exist in disaster-affected populations are, in part, the results of *structural injustices* pertaining to social and economic interactions as well as power relations between agents (both individual and collective) that can be observed at the domestic and international levels. These structural injustices are part of the context in which disaster response is carried out and contribute to how individuals and communities

197

are affected by disaster. The enterprise of humanitarian assistance does not simply occur against the backdrop of these injustices, it is also inextricably enmeshed in these interactions. At the same time, humanitarian assistance following disaster must prioritise among and respond to current health and other needs of survivors, as well as focusing on rebuilding and reconstruction. Our aim in this paper is to offer an improved theoretical account of aid that can help orient humanitarian agencies in understanding and responding to various sources of health vulnerability in disaster-affected populations, with particular attention to questions of justice in the international response to natural disaster.

In our analysis we also draw upon two current avenues of discussion in the field of humanitarian assistance: the denaturalisation of natural disasters and a more integrated conceptual approach to disaster response spanning the traditional categories of relief, reconstruction and development.[2] These ideas are examined and presented in the first section of this paper. In the second section we examine two theoretical approaches for orienting priority setting and questions of justice in aid-programming, an ethics of catastrophe and the social determinants of health model, and discuss their respective strengths and weaknesses for application in this context. We then propose an intermediary approach, *structured health vulnerabilities*, that seeks to integrate aspects of these theoretical approaches, and draws on the works of Paul Farmer and Iris Marion Young with the goal of articulating an account that foregrounds the political dimensions of humanitarian assistance, emphasises the importance of pre-existing vulnerabilities and injustices, and also orients response to pressing health needs.

As we will describe in the following sections, there is often a tension in humanitarian medical assistance following disaster between the need to save lives and provide rapid and efficient care to those affected by disaster, and the need to address root causes of vulnerability. Structured health vulnerabilities bring to attention that an exclusive focus on either of these objectives is problematic. Underlying vulnerabilities and injustices should be factored into operational choices throughout the disaster response process. Failing to do so may exacerbate health issues for the community. However, this assertion does not obviate the need to prioritise saving lives imperilled by catastrophic events, since the outcome of vulnerabilities in a disaster are often acute injury and life-threatening circumstances. Structured

health vulnerabilities in the context of disaster bring into focus the necessity of integrating current acute needs of the ill or injured, as well as inequalities and determinants of vulnerability that shape current and future needs.

1. HEIGHTENED ATTENTION TO DISASTER VULNERABILITY: TWO CURRENT AVENUES OF DISCUSSION

1.1 The Need to Denaturalise Disasters

Social, cultural and political conditions shape the effects of disasters. This reality is less apparent if disasters, and their consequences, are thought of as purely accidental or natural phenomena. It is in line with this observation that commentators have called for 'denaturalising natural disaster' (O'Keefe 1976). As Pinto describes in relation to the Haiti earthquake, 'What is considered natural in the context of disasters such as Haiti's, is seen as independent of human actions. Any analysis of such events must *denaturalise them* by examining the historic, political and economic contexts within which they occur' (Pinto 2010: 193). Pinto warns against well-intentioned but naïve international humanitarian efforts that are not informed by a broader analysis of the pre-existing social, political and historical causes of countries' relative vulnerabilities which often *are* the root causes of disaster vulnerability: 'Without such an understanding, the humanitarian impulse informing the international efforts to support Haiti's recovery and development may serve to merely reinforce the historic relationship between wealthy countries and Haiti and may fuel continued underdevelopment' (Pinto 2010: 193). This process will bring to attention the ways that humanitarian action is itself a product of and contributor to relationships of power and dependence that foster vulnerability.

Denaturalising natural disasters helps respond to another critical question raised by actors involved in relief work regarding the tension between treating acute needs and seeking to address root causes of vulnerability (Bell and Carens 2004). The focus of much humanitarian assistance addresses only the most acute symptoms of a disaster. The principle of humanity directs humanitarian NGOs to focus their efforts to save the lives of individuals affected by catastrophe. In these settings, relief organisations face difficult operational choices in deciding how far to extend their work beyond providing emergency food, potable water,

shelter and healthcare, and address structured health risks that expose the community to greater likelihood of being destabilised by crisis. For example, decisions to design projects in ways that enhance local capacity and resilience within the healthcare sector will have longer-term benefits for the community. Denaturalising natural disasters suggests that questions of vulnerability and inequality should be accounted for as early as possible in the response to catastrophe, without neglecting the importance of providing urgent assistance to those who are in jeopardy.

A further implication of denaturalising disasters is the need to assess the international dimensions of structural injustice that lead to structured health risks within a society. In the field of international ethics, there is a growing literature studying the complex web of inter-relations between macro political and economic structures set at the international level and the domestic conditions of political and economic development within the national sphere. In many crucial respects, unequal political and economic relations between states that are reproduced within transnational institutions (such as the International Monetary Fund or the World Trade Organization, for example) will have a determinant effect on a country's effective opportunities for economic growth and political emancipation (Pogge 2002). This 'globalised' analysis of the co-dependence of international macro-structures and national conditions of economic and political development does not deny the domestic responsibilities of national governments. However, it does highlight the fact that the economic and political vulnerability of some countries is conditioned by the structural interdependence brought about by historical legacies of colonialism and by current unjust forms of political and economic dominations in the international sphere. By economic and political vulnerability, we mean the lack of necessary resources and infrastructure that leaves countries and populations exposed to greater risks of political instability and vulnerability to the impacts of disaster. When catastrophes strike, international NGOs step in. Humanitarian medical assistance following disaster is directed toward helping individuals in need (rather than to fix unequal relations of power between states). Indeed, medical NGOs cannot fully assume the redistributive functions of a national government nor resolve all inequalities within a population. A broader analysis of the international context must still be undertaken to examine the questions of justice that humanitar-

ian medical NGOs confront in disaster response. As Diaz pointedly describes: 'The earthquake revealed our world in other ways. Look closely into the apocalypse of Haiti and you will see that Haiti's problem is not that it is poor and vulnerable – Haiti's problem is that it is poor and vulnerable at a time in our capitalist experiment when the gap between those who got grub and those who don't is not only vast but also rapidly increasing. Said another way, Haiti's nightmarish vulnerability has to be understood as a part of a larger trend of *global inequality*' (Diaz 2011). In this regard, health disparities during and after humanitarian crises point back to pre-existing vulnerabilities both at the national and international level.

1.2 A More Integrated Conceptual Approach to underpin Phases of Disaster Response

Denaturalising natural disasters is also consistent with resisting the tendency to make clean divisions between phases of relief, reconstruction and development, at least at the conceptual level. Dividing disaster response into phases has operational value in that it allows for specialisation of humanitarian actors. These categories make clear that different stages of disaster response require particular skill sets and knowledge bases, as well as distinctive operational priorities, and allow for NGOs to develop expertise in specific areas. However, the theoretical approaches that underlie these activities may benefit from clarifying what unifies them rather than simply focusing on what distinguishes and divides them. A key component that unifies these phases is the role of vulnerability and inequality.

In all phases of disaster response, the determinants of vulnerability and longer-term impacts of aid are important considerations.[3] Following an acute disaster such as a large earthquake, efforts to 'save lives' are the primary focus of humanitarian actors in the initial days and weeks. However, as Pinto argues in the case of Haiti, 'the focus on the immediate humanitarian response appears to have prevented a consideration of how the groundwork for future development could be best laid' (Pinto 2010: 194). Paul Farmer describes how a narrow focus on disaster relief may mask the background and a sub-set of priorities relevant to the situation that hold important consequences for the population over the long term: 'The earthquake was what doctors would refer to as an acute-on-chronic event: a disaster in a setting of profound social precarity' (Farmer 2011a). The acute-on-chronic description helps make clear that addressing acute needs without considering pre-existing vulnerability is mistaken. This perspective is brought into focus in the early stages of disaster response by a unified theoretical approach that crosses over phases of relief, reconstruction and development, and emphasises the role of vulnerability.

The report of the Tsunami Evaluation Coalition, written by Buchanan-Smith and Fabbri in 2005 (Buchanan-Smith and Fabbri 2005), suggests that the phases of Relief, Rehabilitation and Reconstruction are best understood as interlinked and overlapping. While the emergency relief stage is characterised by the immediate concern of saving lives, aspects of longer-term sustainability are still pertinent. Many operational choices have lasting implications for local communities. For example, NGOs can implement programmes in ways that are isolated from local actors or they can seek to build part-nerships and develop local capacity. Relief and rehabilitation should be designed in ways that address needs of vulnerable groups such as the disabled (Wolbring 2011). Thus, both hospitals that are rebuilt fol-lowing a disaster, as well as the design of refugee camps, should be constructed to promote accessibility for and inclusion of people with disabilities. In many ways, this more integrative conceptualisation of disaster response offers opportunities for clarifying how vulnerabilities should be factored into humanitarian medical assistance. It is consist-ent with Farmer's argument that all humanitarian medical assistance should include a broader understanding of the social determinants of health, and should aim to respond to a community's needs and self-determined goals, and design programmes to promote sustainability (Farmer 2011a).

Denaturalising natural disasters and promoting a more integrated conceptual approach to disaster response help focus attention on social vulnerabilities to disaster. However, a challenge in integrating these developments for practice is providing a corresponding theoreti-cal approach for understanding how they relate to the responsibilities and obligations of humanitarian actors in responding to questions of justice and inequality. In the following section we present two theoreti-cal approaches that have currency in the context of disaster response, an ethics of catastrophe and social determinants of health. These approaches emphasise divergent perspectives that roughly correspond with the logics of relief and of development respectively.

2. TWO THEORETICAL APPROACHES FOR DISASTER RESPONSE

The Ethics of Catastrophe

Catastrophes are by definition sudden and exceptional events that cause extensive damage and destruction. Catastrophes, such as natural disasters, suspend normal life and transform responsibilities and roles: different expectations are created for individuals, groups and institutions. Decision-making and the focus of attention of actors are often directed toward immediate needs, including life-saving interventions, with less consideration for longer-term impacts of these actions. An important consideration in catastrophes is maximising benefits across a population. Processes of sorting, prioritisation and allocation are necessary to optimise efforts to respond to a catastrophic event when resources are overwhelmed by the population's needs. Medical triage in mass casualty events is a paradigmatic case. Utility is not the only consideration in the ethics of catastrophe, however. Life-saving may be viewed as having special moral value and thus influence prioritisation away from purely utilitarian approaches.

Two considerations that are particularly relevant to the life-saving goal of disaster relief efforts are the rule of rescue and the humanitarian imperative. The rule of rescue describes a sense of immediate duty to prioritise assistance to identifiable people whose lives or bodily integrity are at risk, without considering the cost expended to save these individuals (Jonsen 1986). The rule of rescue offers a justification for expending resources on providing immediate care to those injured by a disaster even if the aggregate benefits from using resources might be higher if devoted to helping more people with less grave injuries or preserving resources to be used in the reconstruction period. Providing aid to those injured by a catastrophe, even if this aid could lead to more benefit if used in non-disaster situations, may be viewed as morally important. Powers and Faden argue that the provision of aid to communities affected by the Indian Ocean tsunami in 2004 was a matter of justice and that prioritising this aid was justified because of the catastrophic nature of the tsunami: 'Even if it were the case that the global public health responses to this extraordinary tragedy would have produced more QALYs [quality adjusted life-years] had they been deployed elsewhere in the world, to have done so would have been profoundly unjust and not merely unseemly or lacking in compassion' (Powers and Faden 2006). This assertion reflects a view that 'extraordinary tragedies' – catastrophes – should be prioritised even if the response to them is not the most efficient use of resources.

A second consideration that is relevant for disaster situations is the principle of humanity and the related concept of the humanitarian imperative. The principle of humanity is defined as the call 'to prevent and alleviate human suffering wherever it may be found' (International Federation of Red Cross and Red Crescent Societies 1965). It is taken a further step in the Code of Conduct for the International Red Cross and Red Crescent Movement and NGOs in Disaster Relief (RC/NGO Code of Conduct) by the articulation of the 'humanitarian imperative' (International Federation of Red Cross and Red Crescent Societies 1994). The humanitarian imperative asserts the right of access for humanitarian purposes to individuals and populations affected by disaster and in need of assistance (The Sphere Project 2000).

The intersection of the concepts of utility maximisation, public goods, the rule of rescue and the humanitarian imperative raises a number of questions. It is unclear how utility should be balanced off by a priority for emergency response to save lives. Another question relates to the sustainability of humanitarian initiatives, and the long-term consequences of assistance. For example, a beneficiary of aid in Sierra Leone poignantly asks this question: 'You save my life today but for what tomorrow?' (Anderson 2003). This reflection is particularly important in the context of disaster response in situations of underlying instability and poverty.

As discussed above, the ethics of catastrophe describes the distinctive characteristics of a familiar conception of humanitarian assistance deployed in emergency situations in low-resource settings and that is driven by concerns of cost–benefit optimisation and the imperative of saving lives. However, we argue that medical humanitarian assistance cannot solely be guided by the ethics of catastrophe, since this narrow view of disaster relief is unlikely to integrate an analysis of antecedents or include careful attention to likely long-term consequences. Since the ethics of catastrophe are primarily guided by considerations of maximising utility and prioritisation of life-saving interventions, there is limited room for a perspective that looks to the past when the context and origins of the crisis – and collective vulnerabilities – are considered or a future-oriented perspective in which future causes of health vulnerabilities are addressed. In these respects, the following approach seems to overcome some of these shortcomings.

Social Determinants of Health

A second theoretical approach for orienting priority-setting and the focus of medical humanitarian assistance is the social determinants of health (SDH) model. Where the ethics of catastrophe reflects the logic of acute relief, the SDH model is more closely associated with the logic of development assistance. According to the SDH approach, health inequalities are not reducible to *access* to medical care but must rather be framed within a larger political and socio-economic context.[4]

> [P]oor health and health inequalities across individuals and social groups are brought about by multiple and multi-level factors that interact in complex ways. These factors include the individual material circumstances in which people live their lives as well as social cohesion and psychosocial, behavioral, and biological factors, and the functioning of the health care system. The way people interact with or experience these factors is determined by their position in the social hierarchy along dimensions of wealth and income, occupation, education, gender, race or ethnicity, and geographical location of residence. All these causal factors are in turn affected by a political, economic, social, and cultural context that determines the unequal distribution of power, prestige, and resources. (Venkatapuram, Bell and Marmot 2010)

According to this view, systematic gradients of health between groups of individuals (along the lines of ethnic, gender and socio-economic divides) are not reducible to sheer fortune, cultural preferences or individual behaviour. Empirical data on the sources of inequalities are consistent with Daniels' claim that the problem of health inequalities leads to questions of social justice: 'But even if more work is needed to clarify the exact mechanisms, it is not unreasonable to talk here about the social "determinants" of health' (Marmot 1999). To the extent that these social determinants are socially controllable, we clearly face questions of distributive justice' (Daniels 2008). In this way, SDH provides an explanatory model that accounts for vulnerabilities to disaster and draws attention to questions of social justice. Because crises exacerbate health inequalities between groups within a society and between populations in the international sphere, the SDH approach helps us better conceptualise the importance of articulating health needs and social justice concerns beyond the humanitarian imperative and the rule of rescue that characterise the apolitical approach of the ethics of catastrophe.

However, we consider the SDH approach to have important short-comings for offering a comprehensive conceptual approach for the domain of disaster response. The application of SDH for medical humanitarian assistance is limited in at least two important ways. First, while the SDH approach offers a relevant explanation of vulnerabilities, it does not offer an explanation as to how to respond to or prioritise the acute health needs of members of a population that has experienced disaster. Ultimately, there is a risk that if an SDH approach was pri-oritised in aid-planning and resource allocation it could run counter to the humanitarian imperative itself. Instead of a narrow focus on relieving acute suffering without attention to underlying vulnerability (as an extreme version of the ethics of catastrophe might encourage), an unyielding SDH approach would prioritise addressing determinants of vulnerability over responding to acute health needs. Placing abso-lute priority on interventions that address social determinants to the exclusion of addressing pressing health needs might result in a form of 'public health nihilism' (Fairchild and Oppenheimer 1998): for example, digging new wells but not treating individuals already affected by an acute outbreak of cholera, where determinants are addressed but not current health needs shaped by those determinants.

Furthermore, emergency situations in contexts of acute disaster are usually characterised by the partial breakdown or collapse of gov-ernmental structures. In these contexts, not only the humanitarian imperative and the rule of rescue are warranted moral duties, but they might also be the primary ones that medical NGOs can address due to the urgency of the situation and the lack of governance structures. It is important to stress here that while duties of distributive justice incumbent to government are crucial to carry out a full account of the SDH model, NGOs cannot substitute themselves for failed states and assume core governance functions. For example, only governments can use redistribution of income taxes to reduce the impact of socio-economic gradients of health. The SDH model highlights ways in which humanitarian interventions have effects over the long term on recovery, dependence and capacity-building, and is largely compatible with disaster response from the reconstruction through development phases. This model, however, is insufficient to guide a complete account of humanitarian medical assistance. Hence, the need to present an intermediate theoretical approach of humanitarian assistance that integrates aspects of both ethics of catastrophe and SDH approaches.

3. AN INTERMEDIARY APPROACH: STRUCTURED HEALTH VULNERABILITIES

Our goal is to offer an improved account of medical humanitarian assistance spanning the operational phases of humanitarian response to disasters. We propose *structured health vulnerabilities* as a theoretical approach that 1) seeks to enlarge the conceptual analysis, as well as the temporal scope (toward both past and future), of humanitarian relief beyond the ethics of catastrophe, and 2) is inspired by ideas from the SDH model, but attempts to avoid the limitations of the SDH model for disaster response while integrating considerations of social justice into the analysis of the causal factors of certain forms of vulnerabilities. In developing this analysis, we have elected to use the term 'vulnerabilities' instead of 'inequalities' of health. Vulnerability emphasises a dynamic process of marginalisation or exposure to risk. The definition of 'vulnerability' that we employ was articulated by Samia Hurst for the context of health policy and health research and designates 'an *identifiably increased likelihood of incurring additional or greater wrong*' (Hurst 2008).

Hurst directly links vulnerability to the forms and likelihood of harm: 'In order to identify the vulnerable, as well as the type of protection that they need, this definition requires that we start from the sorts of wrongs likely to occur and from identifiable increments in the likelihood, or the likely degree, that these wrongs will occur. It is limited but appropriately so, as it only applies to special protection, not to any protection to which we have a valid claim' (Hurst 2008). By interpreting Hurst's arguments somewhat more broadly, this definition of vulnerability can help to justify special forms of protection and prioritisation for those who are vulnerable in the context of humanitarian health response, and that correspond to the types of limited interventions that are provided by NGOs in disaster settings. In contrast to the social determinants of health model that has been elaborated in the domain of public health, such as taking for granted the existence of a basic institutional structure guaranteed by a minimally functional national government, an approach centred on structured health vulnerabilities is intended for application in situations where governance structures are strained or fractured due to a disaster, and for actors (individuals, NGOs or others) that offer assistance to governments that have collapsed or are badly damaged and are incapable of assuming a governance role. We acknowledge that medical NGOs cannot assume the full range of distributive functions of an autonomous government to address the complex, multifaceted causes of social injustices leading to unjust health inequalities. In short, the structured health vulnerabilities approach is explicitly tailored for non-governmental actors, and takes into account the particular nature of their actions and moral dilemmas in the context of *catastrophe*, as well as the particular constraints that determine the allocation of scarce resources in situations of humanitarian crisis. However, our approach borrows from the social determinants of health model the crucial idea that these vulnerabilities are *structural* in the sense that they are determined by larger socio-economic and political forces that must be taken into consideration even in contexts of acute emergency.

The structured health vulnerability approach also draws on theoretical and practical perspectives introduced by Paul Farmer, which we seek to integrate with certain ideas from the work of Iris Marion Young. Farmer identifies links between social determinants of health and structural forms of injustice (Farmer 2005). He argues that the deprivation of basic needs and human rights violations, starting from the violation of the most basic right to survive, is the pathogenic effect of unequal and unjust power structures both within a particular society and internationally. In Farmer's words, '*the pathogenic role of inequity*' determines the '*structural violence*' (such as human rights abuses) that are linked to the causes of '*structured health risks*'. Farmer argues that 'the social determinants of health outcomes are also, often enough, the social determinants of the distribution of assaults on human dignity' (Farmer 2005: 19). Farmer's analysis of the social determinants of health risks can further propel medical humanitarian assistance beyond the apolitical view of the 'ethics of catastrophe' and toward an approach that attends to the political dimensions of disaster response. If Farmer is right that the health and human rights paradigm should not be confined only to civil and political rights, but must be linked to the 'struggle for social and economic rights as they are related to health' (Farmer 2005: 6), then this is the kind of more comprehensive approach to medical humanitarianism that we want to defend in this paper.

In a number of ways, Farmer's notion of 'structural violence' can be linked to the concept of 'structural injustice' that Iris Young developed, albeit in another context (Young 2007). Young distinguishes the types of injustice that are the result of direct action perpetrated by identifiable agents, who are therefore clearly accountable for the harms that they commit, from structural forms of injustice where the causal responsibility is more collective and diffuse, and thus more difficult to pinpoint. This second type of causal responsibility rests on what Young calls *the social connection model of responsibility*. In this view, there are clear cases of harm whose perpetrators are not easily identifiable. Such harms are the products of complex webs of interactions, from social connections among self-interested agents pursuing their own agendas within common structures (such as economic, political, legal). No one is directly responsible for the harms suffered by those who are most vulnerable to these structural factors. However, to the degree that these harms are the product of the ensemble of social interactions, no one involved can be completely morally exonerated either.

The 'structured health vulnerabilities' approach that we propose points to a model of social connection in order to discern the type of causal role that the international community plays in the production and perpetuation of certain forms of health vulnerabilities. This does not bring into question the fact that in many cases health vulnerabilities characterising certain demographic groups and/or populations can be directly attributed to specific causes and identifiable agents (for example, their own governments). But one of the important implications of our account is precisely to deconstruct the myth that health vulnerabilities are *always* the *exclusive* responsibility of the individuals themselves, and/or corrupt and inefficient members of their own government. In the context of disasters, this suggests that certain health vulnerabilities seemingly caused by 'accidents of nature' are actually shaped by a socio-political context that surpasses the national level. We are not looking to 'prove' the thesis of the causal responsibility of the international community in the genesis and perpetuation of inequalities across the world (following Pogge's work, for example), but rather to argue that a theoretical approach to disaster response needs a scope of inquiry large enough to include the global context of structured health vulnerabilities (in which consists our backward-looking analysis), in order not to reinforce these vulnerabilities in the future (in which consists our forward-looking scope). In this regard, the social and health impact of actions taken by actors in humanitarian medical assistance also needs to be included in this social connection model of responsibility.

At minimum, international assistance should seek not to reinforce pre-existing inequalities nor contribute to future inequities. This assertion is consistent with the view that relief operations should be organised with attention paid to medium- and longer-term implications, and should neither compromise the goals of development nor be complicit in creating or perpetuating inequities (for example, aid agencies should not accept discrimination along ethnic or religious lines in how aid is distributed by partnering organisations) (Ramesh 2008; Malik 2011). Catastrophes reveal the types of vulnerabilities faced by certain demographic groups, as is illustrated by the example of women and children in certain regions of the globe devastated by armed conflict or absolute poverty.[5] 'Conditions in most refugee camps are, to say the least, harsh. Where security is at risk, women, children and the elderly are the most vulnerable. Unaccompanied women in camps can find it hard to secure shelter, adequate food and water rations, medical care and protection from physical and sexual violence (Djeddah 1995; Olness 1998; Allotey and Zwi 2007). Children, who mostly rely on female care-givers, are particularly at risk from malnutrition, as well as violence, abduction into militias and disease due to malnourishment and poor immune defence (Toole and Waldman 1993; Olness 1998)' (Davies 2010: 90). Similarly, minority groups, those who are ill and those with disabilities are likely to experience heightened vulnerability following disaster.

The situation of women in the context of disasters clearly highlights these issues. Documented cases (Enarson et al. 2006) indicate that the types of health risks encountered by men and women differ in the context of humanitarian crises due to socio-cultural features of particular societies: 'Gender relations as well as natural disasters are socially constructed under different geographic, cultural, political-economic and social conditions and have complex social consequences for women and men' (Enarson and Dhar Chakrabarti 2009). In situations of crises, women are more exposed to sexual violence (the location of latrines in refugee camps, for example, is a crucial safety issue), their mobility may be reduced (due to the limited mobility of those they take care of), their health may be at further risk during pregnancy and their economic situation may be extremely compromised. In line with our theoretical approach, the implications for disaster relief programmes and policies should be backward- and forward-looking, while attending to urgent needs for all. 'Pre-disaster activities such as hazard mapping and vulnerability analysis' should take into account gender considerations (WHO 2002). Gender bias (even in the name of cultural values) should be challenged as part of a structured health vulnerabilities approach in aid programming and practice. There is a strong argument for challenging, for example, the introduction of gender into surgical triage as described by a Canadian clinician involved in a humanitarian project: 'It was, "the men are the ones who we need so the men go first to surgery." It was very, very difficult . . . and that was very difficult on the surgeons as well, because they had no say in who, who was to go into surgery first' (Schwartz et al. 2010).

As we have argued, humanitarian actors are also participants in the political economies and political realities that shape disasters and their aftermath. The activities of humanitarian NGOs constitute an influential aspect of the global political and social order. Some organisations have annual budgets that rival those of the states to which they bring assistance (Barnett 2005) and have political influence on a global scale. At the national and local levels the power of NGOs can be significant.[6]

There is thus a need to question the presumption that medical relief can be thought of as an independent activity that can be separated from its larger social context. Such a view, associated with 'classical apolitical humanitarianism' (Weiss 1999), is characterised by a narrow definition of the humanitarian imperative that does not intersect with the analysis of the social causes of pre-existing and future *health vulnerabilities* (encompassing health inequalities and healthcare deprivation). By contrast, recognition that the impact of natural disasters can be correlated to socio-economic and political causes of past, present and future health vulnerabilities suggests that a more comprehensive approach to humanitarian medical assistance is necessary.

CONCLUSION

In this paper we have examined the implications of addressing structured health inequalities and vulnerability in disaster response. This analysis draws on two current avenues of discussion – the denaturalising of natural disasters and a more integrated approach to understanding disaster response spanning the phases of relief, reconstruction and development. This process involves acknowledgement of, and engagement with, the political context of humanitarian crises at local, national and international levels, and a more comprehensive approach to humanitarian programming including attending to longer-term consequences of humanitarian relief. We examined theoretical approaches that can help support this understanding of disaster response, including an ethics of catastrophe and the social determinants of health, concluding that both had strengths and weaknesses. We sought to articulate a third approach, structured health vulnerabilities, that reconciled strengths of the previous approaches and described implications of this approach for humanitarian medical assistance.

Notes

1. We wish to thank Catherine Olivier and Christopher Bourne for their helpful assistance. This paper is part of a research project funded by the Canadian Institutes of Health Research.
2. We distinguish the use of these categories for operational purposes by humanitarian NGOs and the sharp conceptual distinctions that are sometimes drawn between these phases of disaster response.
3. For example, throughout the spectrum of disaster response, actors should be aware that assistance could lead to dependency and hinder local recovery efforts. Harvey, P. and Lind, J., 'Dependency and humanitarian relief: A critical analysis', *Humanitarian Policy Group Report 19*, 2005.
4. In this paper, we do not address the complex philosophical question whether particular health inequalities are *unjust*. For our purposes here, we accept evidence offered in the SDH and public health literatures that demonstrates that *systematic* health inequalities exist between socio-economic and demographic groups within societies and between populations of different countries, which are attributable to the complex interactions of social factors.
5. See Straehle in this volume on instances of vulnerability.
6. Redfield describes how the work of MSF in certain settings takes on an attenuated form of sovereignty (2005).

Chapter 12

'ILLEGAL' MIGRANTS AND ACCESS TO PUBLIC HEALTH: A HUMAN RIGHTS APPROACH[1]

Phillip Cole

1. INTRODUCTION

In this paper I ask whether 'illegal' migrants have a right of access to the public health systems provided by nation-states as part of the welfare provision for their citizens. The answer will have something to do with whether we can establish that they have a right to health which states are obliged to meet. I will argue that they do have such a right, and that right must be met through access to public health systems regardless of 'legal' status. The argument has two parts: first, that the level of agency that should be enjoyed by all human beings, regardless of their 'legal' status, requires that they have access to a certain level of healthcare as of right, otherwise we deny them their full human- ity – we cannot deny people full humanity simply because they do not enjoy full citizenship; second, that those states that have signed and ratified certain international instruments regarding the right to health are obliged, under those instruments, to provide public healthcare to all within their territory, regardless of status, and are in breach of their international obligations if they fail to do so. And so the argument has two aspects: the first ethical, the second legal.

The failure of the argument would mean that our welfare obligations, such as public health systems, can be legitimately restricted to members of the state. We may have some very thin duties of care to those who are within the territory, such as emergency health treatment, but even here we may want to say that if the person receiving that treatment can pay for it, they should do so. My aim is to undermine this position by placing the question within the context of human rights and global justice. The broad point I wish to make is that it is a mistake to think that the global justice perspective is always *outward-looking* – the global movement of peoples means that the commitment to global justice can give rise to *internal* as well as *external* obligations, obligations to 'outsiders' within as well as outside the national territory. This implication of global justice has mostly been overlooked, and the case of the exclusion of 'irregular' migrants from access to public healthcare highlights this paradoxical implication.

In Section 2 of the paper I will describe the practical, political background to these discussions – this is not an abstract question, as liberal democratic states are increasingly taking steps to exclude 'illegal' migrants from access to public welfare of all kinds. In Section 3 I will address the ethical aspect, and the legal aspect in Section 4. I will raise strategic concerns about arguments from human rights in Section 5. My conclusions, of course, raise difficult questions for those who believe in the public provision of welfare resources, such that they have the potential to undermine the feasibility of the liberal welfare project. This is a profound objection to the position I outline here, and I will attempt to address it in Section 6.

2. POLICIES OF EXCLUSION

In 2004 the British government took steps to exclude certain groups of migrants – those considered to be present illegally – from secondary healthcare provided under the National Health Service. The legislation was justified in terms of tackling the problem of 'health tourism', where people allegedly visit the United Kingdom expressly to access free health treatment. In arguing for the restrictions in 2003, the then Health Secretary John Reid said: 'If there are bona fide tourists dropping ill in the streets, of course we will do what we have to, but we are not mugs. There is a difference between being civilised and being taken for a ride.' Failed asylum seekers, for example, were 'effectively stealing treatment from the people of this country'. He concluded: 'I am not talking about emergency treatment, matters of life and death. I am talking about routine treatment that causes the people of this country, who are legally and morally entitled to it, to have to wait longer' (BBC News 2003).

This kind of restriction was, in fact, not new. Charges for overseas visitors using the NHS were introduced in 1982, and clarified in 1989 (Refugee Council 2010; Department of Health 2010). NHS hospital services are obliged to establish whether a patient is an overseas visitor, and, if so, charge them for treatment. There are exceptions: where a person is exempt from charges, so are their spouse and children; people on legitimate business trips and their family are exempt; and, most crucially, anybody who has spent the previous twelve months in the United Kingdom was exempt under the 1982 regulations.

However, one of the amendments in 2004 changed this last rule so that only people living in the United Kingdom *legally* for the past twelve months are exempt, and as a result 'illegal' immigrants, failed asylum seekers, visa overstayers and others living in the country without proper authority are no longer eligible and must now pay for treatment (House of Commons Select Committee on Health 2005: paragraph 94). There are still exemptions in these cases: they will not be charged if i) they have a serious communicable disease which is exempt on public health grounds, including TB and all sexually transmitted diseases apart from HIV; ii) they seek treatment in an Accident and Emergency Department; and iii) they require compulsory mental health treatment (House of Commons Select Committee on Health 2005: paragraph 95). Other changes state that where treatment is judged to be immediately necessary to save life or prevent a condition from becoming life-threatening, that treatment must be given prior to determining whether the patient is chargeable; but this must be determined subsequently and the patient advised as soon as possible, and all costs must be recovered (House of Commons Select Committee on Health 2005: paragraphs 96–7).

These kinds of exclusive measures are not isolated to the United Kingdom, of course. Other Western liberal states have taken or are considering similar steps. In Canada, for example, Bill C-49 would enforce repressive measures against asylum seekers, such as excluding them from public health provision (Health for All 2011). This is at a time when there is already concern in Canada that undocumented workers – estimated at between 100,000 and 300,000 – have limited access to health coverage.

A growing number of clinicians working in primary care with migrant and refugee populations are alarmed because they feel that access to health care is increasingly difficult for undocumented and uninsured families. In contrast, health care institutions may focus on what they perceive to be a potential financial burden, while not recognising that this situation may endanger the life and violate the basic rights of individuals and so constitutes an ethical dilemma. (Rousseau et al. 2008: 290)

If the declared aim of these exclusions is to protect public-provided health welfare systems from 'health tourism', then the evidence is that this is a phantom menace. The House of Commons Select Committee on Health, in its Third Report, published in March 2005, focused on the exclusion of failed asylum seekers with HIV. They stated:

It is very important that the UK does not become a magnet for HIV+ individuals seeking to emigrate to this country solely to access free healthcare. However, neither the Department nor any other interested parties have been able to present us with any evidence suggesting that this is currently the case, or that the introduction of these restrictions on free treatment will actively discourage people from entering or remaining in this country illegally. What little evidence exists in this area in fact seems to suggest that HIV tourism is not taking place. (House of Commons Select Committee on Health 2005: paragraph 111)

In February 2010 the Department of Health launched a general review of access to the NHS by foreign nationals. In its response to that document, the Refugee Council states: 'There is no evidence that refused asylum seekers are "health tourists" seeking to take advantage of free medical treatment in the UK, so restricting entitlement to healthcare does not affect the number of asylum applications made each year' (Refugee Council 2010: 5). A study in January 2010 showed that less than a third of asylum seekers and refugees interviewed had actually chosen the UK as their destination; many did not know they were going to the UK until they arrived. Three-quarters had no knowledge of the UK welfare system (Refugee Council 2010: 5; Crawley 2010). A report by the Royal College of General Practitioners had also found 'no evidence that asylum seekers enter the country because they wish to benefit from free healthcare' (Refugee Council 2010; The Royal College of General Practitioners 2009). The assumption being made by public officials seems to be that asylum seekers have the kind of agency needed to seek out free healthcare in this way, to be health 'tourists', an assumption these reports undermine.[2]

The Department of Health 2010 consultation proposes to reinstate free access to the NHS for certain undocumented migrants, those who have been refused asylum but cannot leave the UK and who are in receipt of support from the UK Border Agency. While welcoming the proposals, campaign groups still believe that all refused asylum seekers should have free healthcare. The Refugee Council points out that due to the complexity of the UK's asylum support system, 'there is no clear distinction between refused asylum seekers who are receiving UKBA support and those who are not. Individuals may fluctuate from one category to the other' (Refugee Council 2010: 4). There are significant delays in processing applications, and those who do receive support are often cut off and have to re-apply. Many are wrongly denied support due to the level of evidence they have to provide, and many are unaware they are entitled to support. 'Denying medical treatment as a consequence of slow and unfair administrative procedures is unethical' (Refugee Council 2010: 4). Those who fall out of this classification, says the Council, 'include families with babies and young children, who are also denied free healthcare under the current and proposed regulations. Inadequate healthcare at this age may have life-long consequences' (Refugee Council 2010: 4).

3. THE ETHICAL ARGUMENT

Campaign groups have understandably focused on powerful consequentialist objections to these policies, but in this paper I ask whether we can place concerns about the exclusion of irregular migrants from healthcare in a human rights framework.[3] In this section I look at the ethical dimension of the human rights argument, digging out the profound moral concerns that provide the basis of the human rights approach. This ethical argument has two parts. The first is a necessary negative groundwork, to set out to answer the criticism that health is not the sort of thing one can have a right to. The second is the positive part of the argument, that the moral content of the right to health is such that it grounds obligations on states to ensure that all within their territory must have access to public healthcare regardless of status.

T. H. Marshall has offered a highly influential three-fold framework for understanding rights. The first is made up of civil rights: 'The civil element is composed of the rights necessary for individual freedom . . . and the right to justice. The last is of a different order from the others, because it is the right to defend and assert all one's rights on terms of equality with others and by due process of law (Marshall 1952: 11). For Marshall, the second element is political: 'By the political element I mean the right to participate in the exercise of political power, as a member of a body invested with political authority or as an elector of the members of such a body' (Marshall 1952: 11). And finally there is the social aspect: 'By the social element I mean the whole range from the right to a modicum of economic welfare and security to the right to share to the full in the social heritage and to live the life of a civilised being, according to the standard prevailing in the society' (Marshall 1952: 11).

This third, 'social rights', framework is fundamental to the liberal welfare approach. John A. Hall has identified it as a crucial component of the liberal idea of freedom: '. . . the secure provision of the basic necessities of food and health, the absence of which makes life miserable' (Hall 1988: 184). This provision, argues Hall, goes beyond mere sufficiency – it must supply the power required to enable the individual to choose from a significant range of opportunities, rather than simply fulfil 'basic' needs. The framework of social rights ensures access to the conditions that underpin the capability to be a fully active participator in the other frameworks, the power to be an active and autonomous chooser and doer of one's own lifeplans, and the lifeplans and projects of one's community, and those of the wider national and global community, that is, the power of agency.

However, two philosophical critiques express scepticism about the conceptual status of socio-economic rights – the institutionalisation critique and the feasibility critique (Sen 2009: 382–3). Onora O'Neill typifies the institutionalisation critique, when she argues that there has to be a connection between the right-holder and 'some specified obligation-bearer(s) . . .' (O'Neill 1996: 382). Without that connection the content of such rights must remain obscure – they must be institutionalised if they are to be counted as *rights*. However, O'Neill does hold that socio-economic rights *can* be institutionalised, and the fact is that they are deeply institutionalised in liberal welfare states, with clear duty-bearers in many cases.

The feasibility critique is expressed by Maurice Cranston, when he argues that it may not be feasible to realise socio-economic rights for all. 'The traditional political and civil rights are not difficult to institute. For the most part, they require governments, and other people generally, to leave a man alone . . .' (Cranston 1983: 13). But how can developing nations be required to respect economic and social rights, given their level of development (Sen 2009: 384)? Amartya Sen's reply is that: '. . . if feasibility were a necessary condition for people to have rights, then not just social and economic rights, but all rights – even the right to liberty – would be nonsensical, given the infeasibility of ensuring the life and liberty of all against transgression' (Sen 2009: 384). He also points out that Cranston is mistaken if he believes that civil and political rights consist in simply leaving people alone – many civil and political rights require extensive positive action by governments, for example genuine and inclusive democratic procedures. He concludes: 'Non-realisation does not, in itself, make a claimed right a non-right. Rather, it motivates further social action. The exclusion of all economic and social rights from the inner sanctum of human rights, keeping the space reserved only for liberty and other first-generation rights, attempts to draw a line in the sand that is hard to sustain' (Sen 2009: 384–5).

But even if we accept the view that socio-economic entitlements can be expressed in terms of rights, the question of the right to *health* remains – should it be included within the list of socio-economic human rights? As Jennifer Prah Ruger comments: 'One would be hard pressed to find a more controversial or nebulous human right than the "right to health" . . .' (Ruger 2010: 119). Liberal theorists have concerns about a right to health. John Rawls identifies primary goods as essential components of any life-goal that can be pursued within a well-ordered society, but makes a distinction between social primary goods (liberty and opportunity, income and wealth, and the bases of self-respect), and natural primary goods, '. . . primary goods such as health and vigor, intelligence and imagination . . .' (Rawls 1971: 303). For Rawls, a theory of social justice is concerned with the basic structure of society, as it is this basic structure that distributes primary goods. However, when it comes to the natural primary goods, '. . . although their possession is influenced by the basic structure, they are not so directly under its control' (Rawls 1971: 62). Therefore they fall under the principles of social justice only indirectly. Samuel Scheffler makes a similar point, that health itself is not a suitable subject for a theory of social justice. Social justice is concerned with the question of the fair distribution of resources and health is not a commodity that can be distributed. However, he says, the things people need for a healthy life *are* distributable commodities, and so do fall under the theory: '. . . people are not said to have a natural right to a good health or a good life, for these are not distributable goods. Rather, each person is said to have a right to adequate food, clothing, and medical care' (Scheffler 1982: 153). And so, while a right to health may not be one that can play a role in programmes of social justice, the right to health *care* can. As Julian Le Grand comments: 'Although in one sense it is true that it is impossible to redistribute health, this does not mean that the distribution of health is insensitive to public policy. For it is obviously possible to influence by policy many of the factors that *affect* health, such as nutrition, housing and work conditions, and, of course, medical care itself' (Le Grand 1991: 113).

Liberal theory does, therefore, allow that the question of health can fall under the distributive principles of social justice, in that the resources of health *care* are distributable, and indeed patterns of inequalities in health do correspond with inequalities in healthcare resources (Cole 1998: 169–73). Therefore, if the distribution of resources is framed in the discourse of rights, then there is no theoretical difficulty in having a right to health as part of that discourse: asserting the existing of the right to health does not constitute a radical challenge to the theoretical structure of liberal thought.

The next stage of the argument is to show that the moral content of the human right to health can ground an obligation on states to provide access to public health systems to all within their territory regardless of status. This consists of establishing that it is a *human* right, a right to those conditions necessary for human agency. There is, I believe, at the heart of the human rights approach a conception of what constitutes a recognisably human life, not so much in terms of levels of health and well-being, but in terms of agency. In philosophical discussions of euthanasia a distinction is often made between a biological and a biographical life – one may be biologically alive but lack a life in any significant sense in that one is unable to engage in the formation of a life story: one has *permanently* lost the capability for writing one's own life narrative. Here I would make a similar distinction between being human in a biological sense, and being human in a biographical sense, having a life *story* which is recognisably human, in that it includes the elements we take to constitute human flourishing, including social and political, as well as economic and physical, elements. This is not to say that people who are being politically, culturally, socially or economically excluded are less than human, but it is to say that they lack the conditions for secure access to this kind of life story, the conditions which would empower them to lead lives that express their full humanity.[4] If we recognise the importance of agency, we can say that human flourishing consists not only in the opportunity to have a recognisably human life story, but also the power to *write* that story, to have a say over its content, and indeed the power to *create* it as it goes along. Asserting humanity is a creative process without a fixed and limited end point, and we can now see that at the centre of the human rights approach lies the project of becoming human together, in solidarity with each other, in the sense of asserting and achieving full membership of humanity and enabling each other to lead a recognisably human life story, with the power to be authors of that story.

If I am right that the right to health must be a fundamental human right, then its content will be derived from a conception of human flourishing essential to the achievement of full humanity. Describing the content of the human right to health is an ambitious project. The first step is to look beyond the emphasis on healthcare *resources* that we find in liberal theory. At a deep level, the problem is not so much how those resources ought to be distributed, but what we ought to be distributing in the first place – what counts as a resource for *health*. Ruger comments that the focus on the right to health *care* 'has left scholars silent on the philosophical foundations underlying a right to health' (Ruger 2010: 120). A practical approach to healthcare delivery has to be grounded on a theoretical picture of human mental and physical well-being or flourishing, and the liberal approach has too little to say about these things to be of much help here. Certainly, those theorists who have developed theories of human well-being have looked elsewhere.

Ruger has provided the most recent and most systematic approach to the grounding of a theory of health by drawing on the capability approach as developed by Amartya Sen and Martha Nussbaum, and through Nussbaum, the work of Aristotle (see Yukiko Asada's and Sridhar Venkatapuram's contribution in this volume for further elaboration of the capabilities approach and its contribution to understanding the human right to health). I will not attempt to represent fully Ruger's approach here, or develop a full philosophical grounding for the right to health. However, I do believe that the capability approach connects closely with my concern with the individual capacity to live a fully human life. For Sen, capability is to be understood as an aspect of freedom, an aspect which connects freedom strongly with agency.

Well-being is not the same thing as agency, but Sen does acknowledge that there are connections between them, such that an increase in well-being may enhance agency (Sen 2009: 286–7). As we have seen, the notion of 'agency', and the capacities and capabilities that underlie agency, are central to the human rights approach, and Ruger connects Sen's concern for agency with health and well-being through drawing on Martha Nussbaum's development of the capability approach and the connection she makes with the Aristotelian concern with human flourishing: '. . . the ethical principle of "human flourishing" under-lies societies' obligations to maintain and improve health capabilities. This principle holds that society should enable human beings to live flourishing lives. Flourishing and health are essential to the human condition' (Ruger 2010: 2).

Central to this philosophical conception of human flourishing and well-being, and therefore to the philosophical grounding of the right to health, will be a conception of the capabilities central to human flour-ishing. For Sen, the capability approach to questions of justice assesses 'a person's capability to do things he or she has reason to value' (Sen 2009: 231); the focus is on 'the freedom that a person actually has to do this or be that – things that he or she may value doing or being' (Sen 2009: 231–2). The focus on freedom and agency is crucial, as a welfare 'dictator' could decide and impose welfare outcomes on a population, such that all members enjoy high levels of health and well-being and a wide range of 'functionings', without ever engaging in the process of deciding what sort of life they want to lead.

The challenge for those using the capability approach is either to identify those capabilities central to their concerns – Sen with agency, Nussbaum with human flourishing, and Ruger with health – or to identify the processes through which those capabilities will be iden-tified. Sen does identify 'basic' capabilities around a conception of basic human needs: 'These capabilities are critical because if they are unavailable, most other capabilities are inaccessible. They are essen-tial prerequisites to other capabilities' (Ruger 2010: 57). However, the emphasis in Sen's work and Ruger's approach is on the latter strategy, the importance of processes for identifying which human capabilities are important and valuable within particular contexts. I will not decide between these two approaches here. The important point for now is that we can argue for the central importance of the right to health for a conception of human flourishing, and can begin to derive the moral content of that right by exploring the capability approach. For the purposes of this paper, if the right to health and the capabilities that make up its content are essential for human flourishing then surely no state can deprive any person of the resources that ground that right without violating their access to the means of human flourishing. If 'illegal' migrants are to be recognised as humans with the right to flourish, then their health needs must be met, and to withdraw the resources that meet those needs is a fundamental failure of recognition.

4. THE LEGAL ARGUMENT

In a sense, there is no question that there is a human right to health, because it is established in international law. The right to health is enshrined in various international instruments. According to Article 25 (1) of the Universal Declaration on Human Rights:

> Everyone has the right to a standard of living adequate for the health and well-being of himself and his family, including food, clothing, housing and medical care and necessary social services, and the right to security in the event of unemployment, sickness, disability, widowhood, old age or other lack of livelihood in circumstances beyond his control. (United Nations 1948)

Article 12 of the International Covenant on Economic, Social and Cultural Rights states: 'The States Parties to the Covenant recognise the right of everyone to the enjoyment of the highest attainable standard of physical and mental health.' These steps include: 'The prevention, treatment and control of epidemic, endemic, occupational and other diseases' and 'The creation of conditions which would assure to all medical service and medical attention in the event of sickness' (United Nations 1966).[5]

The general understanding of the right to health embodied in these international instruments is that it is the right to the highest available standard of health. This itself was expanded on and interpreted by the Committee on Economic, Social and Cultural Rights, when it adopted General Comment 14 in 2000. General Comment 14 itself is not binding, and remains an interpretation of the right to health embodied in international law. However, General Comment 14 has shaped the work of the United Nations and other organisations in this field.

General Comment 14 acknowledges that health is a fundamental human right, and includes certain components, which are legally enforceable (paragraph 1). In a similar way to the liberal theorists we examined in the previous section, the focus is not on health as such, but healthcare. The right is not to be understood as a right to be healthy, but the right to healthcare: 'a variety of facilities, goods, services and conditions necessary for the realisation of the highest attainable standard of health' (paragraph 9). But it is not confined to the right to healthcare, but includes the right to 'a wide range of socio-economic factors that promote conditions in which people can lead a healthy life, and extends to the underlying determinants of health, such as food and nutrition, housing, access to safe and potable water and adequate sanitation, safe and healthy working conditions, and a healthy environment' (paragraph 4).

The committee identified four essential elements to the right to health (paragraph 12): 1) Availability: public health and healthcare facilities, goods, services and programmes have to be available in sufficient quantity; 2) Accessibility: these services have to be accessible to all; 3) Acceptability: these services have to be respectful of medical ethics and respectful to the culture of individuals, minorities and communities, and have to be sensitive to gender and age; 4) Quality: these services have to be scientifically and medically appropriate and of good quality.

In practice, nation-states have a tendency to interpret these rights and protections as owed to their citizens, such that they have discretion over whether they are owed to non-citizens within their territory. However, the United Nations regards its charter of human rights and its other conventions as applying to all people regardless of their status, and therefore takes the view that a national government has an equal obligation to respect, deliver and enforce those rights to all people within its territory.

General Comment 14 makes clear that this interpretation of the human right to health is the correct one. The Covenant explicitly proscribes any discrimination in access to healthcare and the underlying determinants of health (paragraph 18). The obligation on states to respect the right to health means 'refraining from denying or limiting equal access for all persons, including prisoners or detainees, minorities, asylum seekers and illegal immigrants, to preventative, curative and palliative health services; abstaining from enforcing discriminatory practices as a State policy; and abstaining from imposing discriminatory practices relating to women's health states and needs' (paragraph 34).

General Comment 14 is clear that: 'Any person or group victim of a violation of the right to health should have access to effective judicial or other appropriate remedies at both national and international levels. All victims of such violations should be entitled to adequate reparation, which may take the form of restitution, compensation, satisfaction or guarantees of non-repetition' (paragraph 59). This means that the measures taken by the United Kingdom government to exclude certain migrants from access to healthcare provided by the National Health Service are a breach of the government's obligation under international law.

5. STRATEGIC CONCERNS

However, how useful is this conclusion? The fact is that unless the right to health is incorporated into national constitutions, the scope of accountability is extremely limited. In the absence of such incorporation, General Comment 14 can only recommend much weaker strategies: 'National ombudsmen, human rights commissions, consumer forums, patients' rights associations or similar institutions should address violations of the right to health' (paragraph 59). What emerges from addressing the question of justiciability – whether international human rights are enforceable through national courts – is that, when it comes to the right to health, migrants and citizens are in the same boat: if it is not embodied in a constitution, neither has a legally enforceable human right to health.

The lesson is that campaigners against the United Kingdom measures need to look elsewhere than at international instruments embodying the right to health for legal protection or remedy. The Platform for International Cooperation on Undocumented Migrants (PICUM) observes that any legal protection for irregular migrants 'requires an innovative application of the European Convention clauses against cruel and inhuman treatment and respect for family life in the national courts' (Platform for International Cooperation on Undocumented Migrants 2007a: 97). Another form of resistance to the exclusions may come from medical professionals who oppose them, and simply refuse to enforce them: in effect, the rules may be unenforceable if enough medical professionals find them ethically unacceptable. In Sweden, open defiance by pediatricians to state policy aiming to exclude asylum-seeking children from medical care if their claim to asylum was denied has resulted in a special state-funded health programme for those children (Rousseau et al. 2008: 292). PICUM has found that 'health professionals working in community, primary and acute care are reluctant to accept national government pressure to preclude vulnerable migrants from the remit of their services' (Platform for International Cooperation on Undocumented Migrants 2007b). Health-workers are volunteering with NGOs such as Médecins du Monde 'to provide for the immediate needs of undocumented migrants'.

The value of the human rights approach may lie in the arguments in the previous section, concerning the moral content of the human right to health, and the need for an ethical vision of human flourishing to underpin that content. This vision, a theory of the human good, is needed to underpin the legal discourse of human rights here. In the first place, the legal discourse is, by itself, not *pragmatically* persuasive: people, including judges making legal decisions, want a moral justification for a right, not a legal one. In the second place, the legal discourse is not *theoretically* persuasive: it needs the foundation of a theory of the human good to connect it with the world of experience. And if the legal language of human rights is a global discourse – as it claims to be – then the theory underpinning it must be global in scope. There are, of course, many challenges in developing a global theory of the human good that has anything but the thinnest content, as we saw from my meagre attempt in this paper, but the area of health and healthcare may be the most fruitful place to start. And so we come full circle, because the international instruments and the documents and reports that accompany them provide a rich resource with which we can begin to build a global theory of the human good.

6. THE FEASIBILITY OBJECTION

There is one fundamental objection to the position I've defended here. The implication of my argument is that the commitment to global justice and human rights gives rise to *internal* as well as *external* obligations on nation-states when it comes to the provision of welfare. However, to open national welfare systems, such as public health, to all within the territory regardless of status, would be to undermine radically those systems and make it impossible to provide them. The argument seems to be that in order to maintain polities and institutions that are distinctively liberal, such as public welfare systems, there has to be a system of controls that restrict access to those systems, otherwise they will be overwhelmed (Woodward 1992).[6] Whether or not this is true – and I am largely sceptical about 'catastrophe' arguments here – I want to draw attention to the moral force of this objection, or rather its lack of it. How can it constitute a *moral* defence of exclusion? It may be that liberal institutions have a distinctive, perhaps intrinsic, moral value, such that we should protect them, but this doesn't settle the question of who has the right of access to them. Indeed, if they are *that* valuable, the case for excluding others from them looks even less morally defensible.

The danger is that this defence of exclusion takes us toward what I describe as the 'liberal realist' position, such that the attempt to construct a *moral* defence is abandoned.[7] I take 'realism' here from international relations theory, as the view that, as the international order is dangerously anarchic, the only rational approach for nation-states is to pursue their self-interest. Realism rejects what it sees as 'moralism' at the international level – the only rational course is to pursue a self-interested amoralism: the national interest is the only standard against which a state can judge its conduct. This is to take a Hobbesian view of the international order, as a dangerous 'natural condition' in which other states must be regarded as potential threats. Morality stops at the national border, and therefore ethical questions concerned with global justice are ruled out as irrational.

Liberal realism takes this Hobbesian view of the world, holding that not only the liberal nation-state but the liberal institutions that make it up, such as the welfare system, have to be protected from dangerous 'outsiders', even if that requires illiberal practices. A liberal democracy cannot sustain a welfare system or other liberal institutions without restricting membership and access. If we believe that certain institutions are crucial for a just liberal order, then we must be prepared to take the necessary steps to protect them, argues the liberal realist, without concern that this 'just' political order only provides justice to an arbitrarily bounded group of people.

However, once we place those institutions in the context of our commitments to human rights and global justice, and realise that these commitments give rise to internal as well as external obligations, we can see that to defend them by seeking to exclude 'outsiders' undermines our moral position. But in the context of liberal realism, we can say that they are *our* institutions and we must have priority of access to them, while *they* must be excluded from them to some degree or other, and we have to avoid theorising the 'we' and the 'they'. This is a brutally realist, self-interested decision, that we as a 'people' are better off with these institutions, and that this 'national' self-interest dictates that questions of international human rights and global social justice be set aside. In other words, we will restrict access to these institutions because we wish to protect them and maintain them, not for any recognisably ethical reason, but simply because they provide us with what we want, and we want to keep it.

This approach has enormous implications for the very idea of liberal theory and the very ideas of universal human rights and global justice. It may well be that the idea of universal human rights and the question of global justice have no place within liberal political theory, because to place national liberal institutions within a global context undercuts their ethical foundations. All we are left with is the defence of our liberal institutions simply because they are the institutions which give us what we want, and we will not sacrifice what we want in the face of the challenge of global poverty and other inequalities. And so it may be that liberal theorists who are looking for a moral justification for some degree of exclusion of 'outsiders' from either territory or welfare and other institutions are left with a liberal realism which constitutes the abandonment of morality and, ultimately, the moral failure of liberal theory.

As it is presently constituted, liberal theory cannot provide a jus-tification for exclusion and remain a coherent political philosophy, but this is not to suppose that we have reached the end of political philosophy. The membership question constitutes the limits of *liberal* political morality, but not the limit of political theory itself. And so the way forward is to imagine a transformed and genuinely cosmopolitan political theory that is liberatory and inclusive. We need to re-imagine citizenship and the nation-state, and to think of new forms of tran-snational belonging, but it seems that this new way of conceiving of the political order requires radical changes in the nature of political theory itself. Our task as political philosophers is not only to imagine the new global order, but also to imagine the new form of radical cosmopolitan political theory that can act as its intellectual and moral foundation.

Notes

1. This paper was presented at the International Studies Association Workshop on Health Inequalities and Global Justice, Montreal, March 2011. Thanks are due to Christine Straehle and Patti Lenard for organising the workshop and inviting me to attend, and to all the other members for their constructive criticism. Special thanks to Anna Drake for her comments as discussant for the paper. These arguments have been developed in two previous papers: Cole (2007), 'Human Rights and the National Interest: Migrants, Health Care and Social Justice'; and Cole (2009), 'Migration and the Human Right to Health'.
2. Christine Straehle pointed out this assumption to me.
3. Campaign groups do, of course, place their concerns and strategies within human rights frameworks, but there are questions concerning the effectiveness of this, which I will examine in Section 5.
4. Christine Straehle suggested this way of understanding the issue.
5. For other international codes in this area, see International Organization for Migration (2005).
6. For the clearest statement of this view, see Woodward (1992), 'Commentary: Liberalism and Migration', in Barry and Goodin (eds), *Free Movement: Ethical Issues in the Transnational Migration of People and of Money*. For a more recent statement, see Miller (2008), 'Immigrants, Nations, and Citizenship'. For a reply to Miller and others, see Pevnick (2009), 'Social Trust and the Ethics of Immigration Policy'.
7. It might be objected that this is to overlook arguments to do with fairness, around who has contributed to welfare systems through work and taxation. In fact, I do not believe such arguments work, but space prevents me from addressing them here. See Cole (2011), 'Open Borders: And Ethical Defense', in Wellman and Cole, *Debating the Ethics of Migration*, pp. 187–92. Thanks to Christine Straehle for pointing out the need for these arguments to me.

Chapter 13

MEDICAL MIGRATION BETWEEN THE HUMAN RIGHT TO HEALTH AND FREEDOM OF MOVEMENT[1]

Eszter Kollar

INTRODUCTION

Medical migration – the mass movement of medical professionals from the developing to the developed world – is widely seen as one of the most profound problems facing health systems in the poorest countries of the world. Skilled health-workers leave high disease burden areas with acute staff shortages in order to serve patients in low disease burden regions, which are already well equipped. The result of medical migration is deepening global inequality in health.

Sub-Saharan Africa is widely regarded to be suffering the greatest crisis in human resources for health, and data suggests that the problem is likely to grow (Dovlo 2007: 42). The brain drain of health-workers escalates the severe health crises in high disease burden regions that already face a critical shortage of health personnel. World Health Organization (WHO) data show that thirty-six countries in Africa do not meet the 'Health for All' target of one doctor per 5,000 people. On average, there are 1.4 skilled health personnel for every 1,000 people, compared to ten in Europe and in North America (World Health Organization 2006: 98). The WHO has estimated that in order to meet the health-related Millennium Development Goals (MDGs) the number of health-workers in Africa would need to triple. Actual trends, however, run contrary to the global policy target. On the one hand, data from OECD countries show that, in particular in the English-speaking high-income countries, 20–35 per cent of the practising doctors are foreign-trained (OECD 2010). In the UK the number of foreign-trained nurses has grown from 12 per cent to 55 per cent over a decade. On the other hand, in some African countries the expatriation rate of doctors is above 40 per cent and could even exceed 50 per cent

(OECD 2010: 4). In Ghana, for example, roughly half of the graduating doctors and a third of the nurses leave each year, and 40 per cent of the medical jobs are unfilled (Buchan, Parkin and Sochalski 2003).

While brain drain has some positive impact due to remittances and skills-sharing, the overall negative balance manifests in diminishing population health and significant economic losses to the training country. Estimates from the International Organization for Migration (IOM) highlight that developing countries spend $500 million each year to educate health-workers who leave to work in developed countries. Are we, as some suggest, facing a case of 'reverse foreign aid' in the form of economic and health subsidies from the poor to the rich?

It is a well-known fact that healthcare is only partially responsible for the health status of a population. So why focus on the health-workers and their international mobility? When it comes to the most vulnerable regions with the lowest life expectancy, the highest burden of disease, and a weak healthcare system, the number of skilled workers able to contribute to prevention or treatment can make a real difference. The African continent is carrying the highest global burden of disease (25 per cent), and has only half of the healthcare-workers necessary for basic health provision. This absolute shortage is exacerbated by a relative shortage of health workforce, due to the fact that major causes of illness, namely maternal, perinatal and nutritional conditions, and communicable disease, are human resource-intensive areas of healthcare. Consequently, the number of health-workers and the services provided by them can make a significant difference to population health (World Health Organization 2006).

Medical migration is increasingly recognised in international policy discourse as one of the most profound problems facing health systems in the poorest countries of the world. Global treaties and international organisations press for policies to achieve worldwide equitable distribution of health workforce (Global Health Workforce Alliance 2008; United Nations Millennium Development Goals 2000). Prevailing international political morality allocates responsibilities to source country governments and urges them to establish measures to retain their health workforce. Where such state capacity is lacking, the responsibility falls instead on recruiting countries to establish and abide by ethical codes of practice to refrain from active brain drain. Some put the blame on the migrating health-workers, who have violated their social contract with the training country (Snyder 2009: 3–7). Despite the urgency of the problem and the intense international debate surrounding it, however, the solution is far from clear.

The relationship between medical migration and human rights has become a central concern in the discussions. On the one hand, the brain drain of health professionals is widely seen as a human rights violation of the source country populations by recruiting countries. Rich nations actively recruiting doctors and nurses from poor and sick regions are violating the human right to health of the poor. On the other hand, the migrants claim their (human) right to freedom of movement. This claim is further supported by two instrumental claims for open borders based on the alleged developmental effects of remittances and of service sector liberalisation.

The normative debate on medical migration, then, points in two different directions. One person's human right to health is in conflict with another person's freedom of movement and professional choice. Proponents of the former advocate limits on medical migration, while proponents of the latter encourage migration. The first task is to unfold the content of these allegedly conflicting claims in the international normative realm. The second task is to clarify the normative considerations at stake and to see in what sense can global health deprivations constitute constraints on medical professionals' freedom of movement.

1. MEDICAL MIGRATION AND THE HUMAN RIGHT TO HEALTH

The right to health as a human right is widely recognised in international documents.

> Article 25, Universal Declaration of Human Rights (UN 1948): 'Everyone has the right to a standard of living adequate for the health and well-being of himself and of his family, including food, clothing, housing and medical care . . .'

> Article 12(1), International Covenant on Economic Social and Cultural Rights (UN 1966): 'The States Parties to the present Covenant recognise the right of everyone to the enjoyment of the highest attainable standard of physical and mental health.'

Constitution of the WHO (WHO 1946): 'enjoyment of the highest attainable standard of health is one of the fundamental rights of every human being'.

As, in part, exemplified by the above references, the core international human rights documents, as well as the scholars and experts, conflict over what is the exact object of the right in question: health, medical care, healthcare, public health or a standard of living necessary for a healthy life.[2] Let me briefly note some concerns. 'Health' seems to be a problematic object to be protected by a right, insofar as there can be no reasonable guarantee that a person will be healthy. Should people be protected from rare disease or genetic condition, or from personal choices detrimental to their health, as a matter of human rights? 'Medical care' seems too narrow, as it only covers a small portion of what is humanly controllable in a person's health status. It only includes medical treatment to already existing ill-health, while it excludes prevention and other relevant factors determining a person's health status. 'Healthcare' or 'public health' might be more useful categories. They include both treatment and prevention, and have a population-wide aim to protect their subjects from a broad range of threats to health, including epidemic crisis, environmental threats, work-related injuries, and so on. It is widely noted, however, that only a part of a person's health status is determined by her access to medical care or preventive care, while the major determinants of a person's health are social factors, such as socio-economic status, race, gender or the extent of inequality in a society (Marmot and Wilkinson 1999). Should, then, the idea of health as a human right include considerations of social justice? There is no obvious answer, and the debate veils a deeper conceptual problem regarding the nature of the right in question and its proper object. In what follows I will elaborate these issues.

The idea of human rights has been dominantly shaped by a natural law tradition, according to which human rights are possessed by people simply in virtue of their humanity. It has been called the traditional or orthodox view on human rights. On this account, human rights are entitlements that belong to people independently of their membership in social and political institutions, and of their cultural, ethnic, religious or racial belonging. Which rights deserve the special status of human rights is derived from an account of what is of fundamental value or interest in human life, what makes human beings human, or a human life worth living. Grounded in such a way, human rights are universally valuable for all human beings in all times and all places.[3]

If, as the traditional view holds, the proper object of a human right is derived from the idea of fundamental human interest, then health (or some standard of it) seems to be a good candidate for special status. Who would deny that every human being has a fundamental interest in being healthy, independently of their racial or ethnic origins and of their cultural or religious beliefs? Health is likely to have been valued in ancient Greece as much as it is today, and it seems just as valuable to the citizens of Iceland as those of Papua New Guinea. When the grounding idea changes, and we substitute fundamental interests with the conditions necessary for agency or a life lived with dignity, the importance of health seems to follow from all of them. Instead, medical care or healthcare are less plausible candidates, as they are merely of instrumental value to health. So far, so good.

However, when we reflect on the duty to protect the human right to health, and potential violations of it, we run into several difficulties. What sort of actions or omissions count as human rights violations, on the traditional account, remains unspecified. Medical recruitment from vulnerable regions, it could be argued, is a human rights violation insofar as it harms people's fundamental interest in health. Recruiting doctors and nurses from world regions that not only desperately need to retain their existing health workforce, but would need to increase it in order to provide the most basic health services, seems to fall under this category, for at least four reasons. First, we are dealing with countries with acute shortages in their health workforce. Second, some of the main forms of illness require human resource intensive care. Third, emigration occurs in large numbers, which can leave entire regions, especially rural areas, without access to medical assistance. Finally, the recruitment of rare specialists may lead to the closing of whole medical departments and leave a country without specialist care. In short, the recruitment of doctors and nurses from vulnerable regions undermines or further diminishes an already weak state capacity to provide basic health services. Despite the complexity and the indirect nature of the causal relationship, medical recruitment is a human right violation due to its consequences for diminishing population health.

The difficulty is that a human right so conceived yields too broad a scope for the actions and omissions that may properly count as human rights violations. Besides recruitment on the part of affluent nations, the poor country that fails to retain its health workforce as well as the migrating professionals are potential human rights violators. According to the traditional account, a just state of affairs is one in which every person enjoys adequate health, and whenever a significant number of people fall below the threshold, human rights violation occurs. Any government action that contributes to diminishing population health below the relevant threshold violates the human right to health. There are, however, many forms of government action or omission that we would hesitate to call a violation of people's human right to health, despite the government's failure to protect people's fundamental interest in being healthy. Among them are failures to prohibit smoking in public spaces or failure to ban unhealthy foods for consumption. If we are reluctant to judge every action or inaction that contributes to diminishing population health to be a human rights violation, there must be something more to the human right to health than our fundamental interest in being healthy.

One way to narrow its scope is by narrowing the relevant kinds of threats the right needs to protect against to 'standard threats'.[4] The human right to health, then, does not need to protect people from all forms of rare or unpredictable disease, but only from reasonably predictable and humanly preventable forms of ill-health. Widespread communicable or nutritional diseases, whose remedies are well known and can be produced and disseminated at a reasonable cost, surely fall under this category. Consider that despite some improvement, in sub-Saharan Africa still one in eight children dies under the age of five, most of them in the first month of life, mainly due to pneumonia, diarrhoeal diseases and birth complications (UNICEF 2011). That is, from diseases that we know are preventable through adequate nutrition and neonatal care. These children, then, have an uncontroversial claim given that their fundamental interest in health (or bare survival) is threatened by a standard threat. For their rights to be meaningfully claimable, however, there is a further element to be added to our understanding of human rights. We need to take seriously the idea of *rights* in human rights and the idea that only those claims can count as human rights that are weighty enough to demand protection and to, thereby, limit other people's freedom. Joseph Raz's critique of the traditional view is particularly helpful here.

According to Raz (2006), the traditional view, and most advocacy groups guided by it, fails to acknowledge the nature of rights in its complexity. It is true, he argues, that rights generally protect things that are of fundamental value to people. However, it is not enough to establish that the object of the right in question is valuable to the right-holder. There are many things we value, and deem fundamentally important to human life, yet do not have a right to. Besides being of value to people, rights, equally importantly, limit other people's freedom. A secure enjoyment of a right pre-supposes that other people have a duty to protect it. As Raz says, 'rights have a special role in our moral universe: they apply to cases where the value of something to a person is of a kind to warrant holding others duty-bound to respect it in some ways' (Raz 2006). A right, then, protects those objects of value that warrant constraints on other people's freedom. So the value it protects must be so special, it must be 'of a kind' to justify other people's obligation to secure it for its possessor. So for something to qualify as a right, it requires a valuable object and the secure enjoyment of it, incorporating the grounds on which other people should protect it. And this is the aspect of rights, for which traditional conceptions of human rights fail to account sufficiently. In fact, traditional theories focus their attention on the idea of humanity, or what is peculiarly human about human beings, in establishing the relevant category of rights. In a way, they highlight the *human* side of the story, and shadow the *rights* side of the story.

Human rights are a special category of rights. They protect things that are of fundamental value to all people under current conditions of life. They must also include grounds that constrain the actions of a particular type of agent, namely nation-states. Human rights are international moral standards that limit state sovereignty, and their violation justifies intervention by outside agents.[5] As Raz concludes, they protect valuable things of a kind sufficient to impose duties on people within and outside state borders and to warrant interference in the internal affairs of a state (Raz 2006). The human right to health, then, must be specified as protecting a fundamental human interest in health from reasonably predictable and preventable common forms of ill-health, whose violation is sufficient to limit the permissible actions of international agents. It seems that mothers in labour and their children whose lives are threatened by insufficient pre- or neonatal care have a reasonable claim that places limits on the permissible actions of international agents.

Add to that a final distinction concerning the type of action that can count as human rights violations. Thomas Pogge has extensively argued (Pogge 2007; Pogge 2002) that agents can be causally related to violating people's human rights in various ways. Most obviously, when they foreseeably and avoidably harm others in their fundamental interest. Call this, after Pogge, an *interactional* human rights violation. The classical example is a river pollution with devastating consequences for the livelihoods of people depending on the river and the surrounding land. Human right violation is an assessment of the polluter's activity that harms the victims. In other cases, inaction or failure to alleviate poverty, rather than active impoverishment, can constitute a human rights violation. Pogge argues that any social order that requires people's co-operation owes them the secure access to their basic necessities in return. Human rights, on an institutional account, are claims on social institutions for a secure enjoyment of their objects. Assuming that there exists a feasible institutional reform under which those deprived could have been better off, governments that rely on their citizens' co-operation to abide by the law and pay their taxes, yet nevertheless fail to meet their citizens' basic needs, share a responsibility in their suffering.

The problem with medical migration from vulnerable regions, then, is the following. Health, a fundamental interest shared by all people, a necessary condition of a decent life, or a life at all, is threatened by preventable diseases. Given the nature of disease, prevention, in part, depends on the presence of a sufficient number of health-workers. Source country governments are, in part, responsible for the process, when they fail to alleviate suffering and when they fail to retain their health workforce, assuming that they could have done otherwise. Governments making bad policy choices that underdevelop health services and undersupply health workforce amounting to health deprivations would fall under the category of human rights violation by omission.[6]

It is, however, much less plausible to blame source countries when the failure to retain their health workforce is due to a weak state capacity. Moreover, the moral case is complicated by the fact that domestic efforts to retain health workforce are undermined by international actions and policies. A major pull factor for medical migration is active recruitment. Recruitment, through a complex causal chain of events, results in health deprivations. The right to health and basic survival incorporates a claim sufficiently weighty to justify interference from outside agents in the form of assistance or aid. Destination countries, however, not only fail to assist those in need, but drain the local sources of assistance, thereby undermining an already weak state capacity to provide basic healthcare. It seems, then, that we are dealing with a case of human rights violation and the case falls under the category of an international 'interactional harm'. The combined actions of agents in one country, recruitment agencies and the government policies enabling them, foreseeably and, most likely, avoidably deprive people in another country of their basic health.

Both accounts of human rights violations, whether due to an action or an omission, require constraints that determine the permissible policies in source and destination countries. Source countries are required to work toward retaining their health workforce, while destination countries should refrain from recruiting doctors and nurses from vulnerable regions. As a 'side-effect' these efforts constrain the freedom of movement of professionals, the migrating doctors and nurses who seek better work and life prospects. The question is whether we can find reasons sufficient for limiting their freedoms. In what follows, the argument for professionals' freedom of movement will be examined.

2. MEDICAL MIGRATION AND THE FREEDOM OF MOVEMENT

Healthcare professionals leave their country of origin for a variety of reasons. The major cause underlying migration is the wage differential between source and destination countries accompanied by opportunities for a better quality of life. Scholars have noted that 'source-destination country wage differentials (adjusted for purchasing power parity) are so large (3–15 times) that marginal increases in source country wages would, alone, not affect migration flows' (Alkire and Chen 2006: 108). In addition to wage disparities, among the main push factors for skilled workers are poor prospects for professional training, poor working conditions, poor living conditions topped with violence, conflict and war, and last but not least, weighty private reasons (World Health Organization 2006).

The arguments supporting open borders policies for medical migration are based on three concerns. First, the migrants themselves claim their right to freedom of movement in order to seek better life prospects (see Christine Straehle's chapter for an elaboration of this argument).

Second, the 'remittances for development' claim holds that benefits from labour migration through private financial flows exceed the development potential of international aid, hence labour migration should be encouraged. Third, the 'free trade for mutual gain' view holds that the liberalisation of health services, that is, when countries open their healthcare system and reduce trade barriers to allow the free flow of goods and professionals, will result in economic benefits for all parties involved. Let us examine these three claims in detail.

Right to Freedom of Movement

The dominant policy solutions on both ends of medical migration point in the direction of limiting professionals' freedom of movement. The main challenge for source countries is how to retain their trained health workforce. Policy measures include education with mandatory service; that is, in exchange for their medical education students have to sign a contract, in which they agree to provide service in their home country for a specified number of years. On the receiving end, destination country governments are under international pressure to introduce ethical codes of practice to refrain from harmful health-worker recruitment.

In response, medical professionals claim their universal human right to freedom of movement. However, the content and requirement of such a right often remains unspecified. Freedom of movement is limited in an obvious way by the existence of state borders and visa restrictions. In what sense is there a human right to freedom of movement, then? Article 13 of the Universal Declaration of Human Rights (UDHR) stipulates:

1. Everyone has the right to freedom of movement and residence within the borders of each State.

2. Everyone has the right to leave any country, including his own, and return to his country.

According to the first paragraph, people who are born in a country or have already acquired entry into a country should be free to move and change their residence within the borders of that state. The second paragraph, instead, stipulates a right of exit and re-entry in one's own country, without any reference to taking up residence or work in a country outside one's own. For a better understanding of the second claim, we need further insight into the international human rights corpus.

Article 12 (§3) of the International Covenant on Civil and Political Rights (ICCPR):

> The above-mentioned rights shall not be subject to any restrictions except those which are provided by law, are necessary to protect national security, public order (ordre public), public health or morals or the rights and freedoms of others, and are consistent with the other rights recognised in the present Covenant.

It is clear from the above passage that there are recognised restrictions on people's freedom of movement in international law; among them are public health and the protection of other human rights. What exactly constitutes a reasonable public health constraint on people's freedom of movement might be subject to disagreement in international legal discourse. Whether it only applies to extreme and urgent cases, such as a quarantine in a pandemic crisis, or can be extended to extreme conditions of a more permanent nature, such as global health deprivations in vulnerable world regions, is still unclear.

Beyond the legal interpretation there is a more pressing normative question. *Should* there be any restriction on people's freedom of movement? Do severe health deprivations in poor countries constitute justified constraints on the right to freedom of movement of medical professionals?

On the one hand, one could argue that the global health crisis and its accompanying human resource crisis together result in such extreme health deprivations in certain parts of the world that the human suffering and the human lives at stake constitute sufficient grounds for limiting medical professionals' freedom of movement. Healthcare-workers, given their special skills combined with local knowledge, are in a particular position to help and ease suffering in a very tangible way, and as such they have a moral obligation to serve (at least for a period of time) the country that trained them. On the other hand, one could argue that it is unfair to place the whole burden of the 'global burden of disease' on a particular group of skilled professionals born into developing countries. What about other skills relevant for poverty eradication and development? Should we place restrictions on their movement too? Or perhaps restrictions should apply to skilled migrants on the whole? The further we go down that road, the more implausible our proposal becomes. Source country restrictions on the freedom of movement of skilled professionals penalise people for pursuing hard educational choices, and could even create adverse educational and professional incentives away from the medical profession toward restriction-free sectors.

Some positions in the debate avoid the dilemma altogether. One could be in favour of professional migration and opt for taxes and other financial measures, through which the medical migrants can repay their brain drain debt to the training country. Let us examine one of the arguments in detail.

'Remittances for Development'

The 'remittances for development' view (Barry and Overland 2010: 1181–207; Barry 2011: 31) welcomes and encourages professional migration from developing countries to developed ones. Its proponents claim that more freedom of movement rather than less would be beneficial to the poor, which, in turn, may have a positive impact on reducing poverty-related ill-health. The claim rests on a concern with global inequalities and feasible development instruments that can reduce the gap between the rich and the poor. Its proponents observe that under current demographic and labour market conditions the developed world is suffering from ageing populations and shortage of workforce, while the developing world is facing overpopulation and high unemployment rates. Unconstrained labour migration, they argue, could even out the shortage of workforce in developed countries with the surplus in the developing world. What is more, remittances are likely to benefit the poor.

Remittances are financial flows between the source and destination countries in the form of private transactions from the migrant to his family or relatives at home. Its private nature is one of its main advantages. Firstly, compared to other development instruments, such as international aid or government-funded projects, it seems to be more efficient in meeting people's needs, due to the sender's direct knowledge of the nature of the need and the family's greater incentive to spend it responsibly. Secondly, the migrants at the benefactor's end have strong motives to care for those left behind (Barry and Overland 2010). These positive private incentives manifest in a remarkable outcome. Studies report that the level of private flows exceeds the amount of international aid or foreign direct investment. As such, it is considered an important financial instrument for development.

Scholars with reservations concerning the effects of remittances on development point to some of its problems (Brock 2009b: 204–10). Without hoping to settle the general debate, a few considerations seem particularly relevant from the point of view of medical migration and population health. First, who are the real beneficiaries of remittances from migration? Which segments of the population benefit from it? This relates to the more general question whether remittances can be considered a pro-poor development instrument. Generally speaking, the least advantaged in developing countries lack the necessary capabilities, education and economic resources for labour migration, hence cannot directly benefit from the private flows (Brock 2009b: 205). Doctors and nurses are skilled migrants who are unlikely to come from the poorest families, while a large portion of ill-health in developing countries is due to conditions of extreme poverty, including malnourishment, bad housing, lack of water and sanitation, and so on. There is likely to be a discrepancy between those segments of the population who carry the highest burden of disease and the households that benefit from remittances. The least advantaged, who are the least likely to migrate and the most vulnerable to disease, are likely to lose out in the process. As remittance sceptics note, medical migration carries serious disadvantages for the country of origin. The populations left behind lose in terms of the investment in education and training of health-workers, and in terms of the healthcare resources and health services (Brock 2009b: 203). Medical migration can leave vast areas, especially rural and unattractive urban areas, without medical assistance, and in the most vulnerable areas can lead to the collapse of the public healthcare system (World Health Organization 2006).

The second question relevant for medical migration is in what way do source country populations benefit from remittances. How are remittances spent by their beneficiaries? What sort of goods do remittances create for source populations? Studies report that households benefit from remittances mainly in the form of private consumer goods. Income received from remittances is largely spent on living expenses and consumer goods, and a small portion of it goes into savings and micro-investments (Brock 2009b: 205–6). This raises the question of whether remittances are good financial instruments for tackling disease and ill-health. While certain elements of ill-health can be improved by private investment alone, such as meeting nutritional needs or purchasing drugs, many aspects of health cannot be maintained or improved without public investment in healthcare, education, living conditions and the environment. Health (care) is a public good, which requires society-wide contribution and co-ordination in order for it to be effective in meeting population needs. Unless part of the private transfers is channelled into public healthcare funding, the effects of remittances on populations' health are likely to be negligible. Those in favour of remittances are more reluctant to assign the state a central role in development, and welcome private means that can empower the citizenry vis-à-vis the government; understandably so, especially when dealing with unaccountable and corrupt governments. It seems, however, that insofar as public goods are concerned, a collective solution can hardly be avoided. Potential revenues for such interventions may come from some form of compensation on the part of the emigrating professionals or the benefiting host countries. Instruments may include educational debt repayment or mandatory service for medical migrants. It has also been suggested that destination countries should pay compensation to the training country after each trained medical personnel recruited (Brock 2009b: 203).

'Free Trade for Mutual Gain'

Economic liberalisation rests on a classical economic thesis, according to which free trade arrangements in goods and services result in more efficient production and exchange from which all parties benefit. If so, then, the liberalisation of trade in health services may result in mutual economic gains for the countries that open their healthcare system to the free movement of goods and professionals. The picture is not so simple, and international trade liberalisation efforts have generated harsh criticism on the part of economists, healthcare professionals and activist networks on human rights and alternative globalisation. Let me, however, point out a few aspects of the debate relevant for our case.

The most influential multilateral agreement affecting medical migration trends is the World Trade Organization's General Agreement on Trade and Services, the main outcome of the Uruguay Round of trade negotiations in 1995. Signatory governments have committed to reducing and removing trade barriers to international exchange and foreign investment in service sectors, among them healthcare. In general, the GATS has rendered national health services vulnerable to global market forces. Regarding professional migration trends, it has facilitated the adoption of active recruitment policies in affluent nations that try to fill their increasing health-worker shortage with foreign-trained health personnel (Bach 2003).

Proponents of health sector liberalisation emphasise how much certain developing countries have benefited from the process. As noted by the latest OECD report, some countries with a high 'percentage of their health personnel abroad manage to maintain relatively high numbers of health workers at home. This is the case notably for countries that train nurses for export, such as the Philippines, some Caribbean states and, increasingly, China' (OECD: 5). By investing in their health system they managed to streamline their health education and to produce a surplus in their health workforce who are now enjoying the advantages of foreign recruitment. Despite these success stories of health sector liberalisation, however, we must be cautious in generalising success.

While some countries are able to turn these trade opportunities to their advantage, many, especially the vulnerable, nations seem to lose out. The entry-level stage of development, in part, explains this discrepancy. On the one hand, a country's bargaining position at a trade negotiation table strongly depends on its stage of development. We have good reason to think that small low-income countries with a weak state capacity are likely to make bad deals. They lack the economic means, knowhow and political power in a global political setting to be equal negotiating partners. Moreover, the populations most vulnerable to disease and poor health often lack democratic control over their governments, and it is rather likely that their unaccountable political elites are negotiating behind closed doors without public control. Even in more democratic settings there is little or no collaboration between trade policies and the health policies, and GATS commitments are made at a fast pace without public consultation or deliberation.

On the other hand, service sector liberalisation renders developing countries with a critically weak health sector particularly vulnerable to global market forces. Critics of health sector liberalisation under the GATS regime note that the 'net economic benefits of trade in health services are at best limited, strongly skewed towards the better off, and come at a high cost in terms of health of the majority of the population' (Woodward 2005: 530). They suggest that health should be taken off the trade agenda, or at least constrained by strong conditions protecting the health and well-being of member country populations.

CONCLUSION

Should we tame or encourage medical migration flows, then? There is no simple answer. The solution requires a sound understanding of its causes, consequences, and the kind of human vulnerabilities that are at stake at the origin and destination ends of the process. What is clear, however, is that prior to settling on any viable policy there are tough ethical choices to be made. Population health and professional freedom of movement are both important values to be protected. Is health, in any way, special that it deserves priority over other worthwhile human concerns? When people's lives are threatened by preventable disease, our judgement pulls toward the priority of health. Then again, how much professional freedom of movement are we willing to sacrifice for the sake of health? The answers require extensive ethical and political deliberation even within a domestic society, and much more so in the global political arena, given the rich diversity of views about the human good, the relative priority of fundamental values, and the emerging nature of global institutions through which such ethical dilemmas could be fairly and effectively resolved.

Notes

1. I would like to thank Patti Lenard, Christine Straehle and Tiziana Torresi for their helpful comments and suggestions.
2. On the distinction between medical care and public health, see for example Mann (1997).
3. See for example Griffin (2008). For a critical analysis, see Raz (2007); Beitz (2009), pp. 49–73; and Wenar (2005), pp. 285–94.
4. This idea is classically articulated by Shue (1996) and recently restated by Charles Beitz as a political conception of human rights. See Beitz (2009), pp. 110–11.

5. This view first appeared in a brief statement on human rights in Rawls (1999) and further elaborated by Raz, 'Human Rights in the New World Order', and Beitz (2009).
6. For an in-depth account, see Pogge (2007).

Chapter 14

HEALTHCARE MIGRATION, VULNERABILITY AND INDIVIDUAL AUTONOMY: THE CASE OF MALAWI

Christine Straehle

Few would argue that access to healthcare is equitably distributed around the globe. Most would instead agree that living in a developed country gives a person more extensive access to healthcare than citizens of developing countries have. The definition of access to healthcare I want to employ here is that a person has access to a health professional like a physician, nurse or midwife when they need to, and that the health professional is able to provide minimal prevention, education and treatment to them.[1] One of the aggravating factors given for inequality in access to healthcare is the unequal distribution of healthcare professionals, very often heightened by migration of healthcare professionals from developing countries to developed countries. Many nurses and doctors from what we may call *health provision poor countries* choose to migrate to other countries to provide services and employ their skills there. This has led to a critical undersupply of doctors and nurses in their source countries, a situation defined by the WHO as less than 2.28 health-workers per 1,000 population, and less than 1.71 nurses per 1,000 (WHO 2009: 15).

In response to detrimental outmigration of health professionals, some have argued that developing source countries should be permitted to at least impose conditions on outmigration by healthcare professionals. The hope is that sending societies will thus be able to recoup some of the costs and burdens they have incurred in training doctors and nurses. Otherwise, the worry is, they might quickly become healthcare *deprived* countries. Such exit restrictions may take different forms: proposed scenarios range from demanding a set time of service in the country of origin after the end of professional training and before enjoying the possibility to emigrate; others suggest that countries should be permitted to levy an 'exit tax' on migrants who have benefited from a system of education but who intend to carry their skills abroad.

A look at actual figures may illustrate the problem best: in Kenya, for example, it is estimated that the cost to educate a doctor from primary school to university graduation amounts to US$65,997, while educating a nurse costs US$43,180 (Kirigia et al. 2006).[2] Compare these figures to those published by the British Medical Association in January 2011, which put the training costs for British doctors between US$436,000 and US$620,500, depending on the level of doctor (BMA Press 2011). It is fair to say, then, that the current situation is a de facto subsidy that developing countries provide to their developed counterparts, by training what are to the latter inexpensive healthcare-workers at a high cost to the former (Kapur and McHale 2006).[3]

The aggressive recruitment of health professionals from health resource poor countries is problematic from a global justice perspective, and helpful suggestions for ethical recruiting procedures have been made (see Brock 2009a). Developed societies that yield the fruits of foreign training of doctors and nurses, thus heightening their already high supply of health professionals, have duties and obligations toward the countries that shoulder the burden of educating doctors and nurses at a high price to them. To satisfy these duties, recruiting countries should pay compensation to the sending country or actively assist in the training of health professionals, for example (see Kapur and McHale 2006).

It is not clear, however, that the moral argument for compensation also supports exit restrictions imposed on individual nurses and doctors. Such measures have been justified from different positions – I will call the first line of argument the *reciprocity* argument; whereas I will refer to the second argument as the *argument from social justice*. The reciprocity argument builds on the just-illustrated facts about the social costs of educating and losing medical professionals. But even without putting a monetary value on the training of the individual, the idea is simply that societies invest in their young through a range of social goods and provisions and that members are under a certain obligation to acknowledge this and 'reciprocate' for the benefits and advantages received. We don't usually accept free-riding behaviour in societies and so it is not clear why we should accept it in the international sphere (see Ypi 2008).

The argument from social justice takes a slightly different form.

According to this line of reasoning, individuals are under obligations to contribute to the welfare of all members of the community in which they were able to train as health professionals if this community is engaged in a project of social justice. Note that this line of justification for exit restrictions only applies to legitimate, democratic states (Brock 2009a). The argument from social justice is not only based on benefits received from the sending society – rather, it appeals to the need to co-operate when realising social justice goals (Rawls 1999; Ypi 2008). Put differently, societies should be allowed to put certain restrictions on individuals in their exercise of autonomy if the unfettered exercise of individual autonomy risks jeopardising the basis of social justice, which in turn provides others with the means for individual autonomy (see Ypi 2008 for a discussion of this argument).

Both of these arguments for restrictions of emigration of health professionals sound plausible for most cases of health-deprived countries if we accept a consequentialist argument: if sending societies invest in healthcare-workers' training at great expense, and these same individuals then move away, it is fair to assume that sending societies suffer. What is not so obvious, it seems to me, is whether or not exit restrictions on the individual professional can be justified from a moral perspective that is concerned with individual autonomy. Such restrictions, in fact, raise a set of questions about how to balance the good they aim to promote – retaining health professionals in the country for the good of the country's population – with the good they would potentially put at risk – the realisation of the individual's life-plan.

To be successful, the moral argument for emigration restrictions (I will stay with this term even though one may debate if an exit tax or imposed period of service in fact represents a restriction, or simply imposes a condition of exit) needs to provide positive links between the following issues: first, it needs to show that the emigration of healthcare-workers represents a moral wrong, and that exit restrictions can be construed as effectively addressing this same moral wrong. Second, it needs to show that imposing exit restrictions is 'morally neutral', which is to say that the restriction does not impede the realisation of a comparable moral good, never mind jeopardising it. It seems to me that at this point in the argument, different scenarios may arise. In the first case, we may find that restrictions indeed help to prevent or rectify a moral wrong; and that they are indeed morally neutral insofar as they don't impede the realisation of an equally valuable moral good. We may then accept exit restrictions on healthcare-workers as justifiable.

Alternatively, we can imagine a situation in which exit restrictions, while helping to avoid moral wrong, are nevertheless not morally neutral. I will propose that this scenario represents a conflict of moral goods – which is to say that the moral good that restrictions promote may be equally valuable and commensurable to another moral good, the realisation of which is put into question or jeopardised by exit restrictions. The goods conflicting as I construe them are the provision of adequate healthcare access in the country of origin on the one hand, and the realisation of a nurse's or a doctor's individual autonomy through a chosen 'migration project' (Ottonelli and Torresi forthcoming) on the other hand.

In this case, we have again two options: first, we may find that the competition between two moral goods needs to be balanced and evaluated carefully. One way of doing this might be to assess the kinds of restrictions proposed, and to evaluate whether or not some pass a test we may devise – what we may call the 'proportionality test' of exit restrictions. We may find that some restrictions can be justified since they don't contravene the pursuit of the competing moral good permanently, while also helping to avoid moral wrong. Or we may find, secondly, that exit restrictions do not pass the proportionality test, which is to say that they can't be justified with their positive effects; that their negative effect on the migration project of the individual is so grave that nothing can justify them. In this case, it seems clear that from a moral perspective, such restrictions on individual autonomy can't be justified.

In the course of this paper, I investigate whether or not emigration of nurses – and I focus here on the case of Malawian nurses – constitutes a moral wrong that may justify exit restrictions (Section 1). I will argue that the moral wrong caused is that of creating heightened vulnerability to harm of some members of the sending society. I will define harm here as dying from diseases that might have been detected and treated if access to healthcare had been available more readily. Specifically, I will argue that such vulnerability derives from the understaffing of many of the country's rural healthcare centres, a situation that leads to diminished healthcare provisions in those areas – particularly a lack of prevention and treatment of diseases that leads to high numbers of maternal and under-5-year-olds' deaths. Assessing the first step necessary to establish the justifiability of exit restrictions outlined above, I construe the moral wrong that the emigration of nurses provokes as in a first instance taking the form of not alleviating and protecting some members of Malawi society against a background condition of vulnerability. I conclude this section by accepting that good arguments can be made for the link between less emigration of Malawi nurses and better prevention and treatment for mothers and children, particularly in rural Malawi.

The moral good I juxtapose to this goal is twofold: in a first instance, emigration can help to improve the means of individual autonomy of those who choose to emigrate. Here I endorse a definition of autonomy that relies on the idea of self-determination and self-realisation of self-set goals in life (Section 2) and explain how for many women nurses in Malawi, emigration provides for better options. Second, I explain that for many nurses emigration allows them to provide for those staying behind.

So on the one hand, emigration induces vulnerability that can lead to harm for some; on the other hand, the same migration promotes individual autonomy of nurses and provides them with the means to provide for their family members. Put differently, emigration is then not only a vehicle for moral wrong – to create heightened vulnerability – but can also serve as a tool for the realisation of a moral good – to realise autonomous goals and to satisfy obligations towards family members.

This leads me to Section 3, in which I try to balance the two goods. Here I argue against a set period of service after graduation. I justify this with the needs among those staying behind, which may be most virulent at one specific point in time, rather than five years later. The exit restriction of a time of service would then not pass the proportionality test. Levying a specific kind of exit tax, on the other hand, could potentially be justified. However, I argue that in order to pass the proportionality test, only a rather low percentage amount of a nurse's salary could be charged. If the aim is to preserve an individual's possibility to realise her migration project that includes providing for close others while also taking into consideration living expenses in her adopted country, then not much will remain to be possibly paid back to the country of origin. Yet then, I conclude, we may wonder what good such a restriction would do besides being symbolic. If the goal is to discourage emigration or to compensate for the loss of a valuable nurse then much higher amounts would have to be raised; the more plausible route to address unequal access to healthcare is to shift the burden onto recruiting countries and require them to pay a 'head tax' to sending countries.

1. WHAT IS THE PROBLEM? VULNERABILITY IN MALAWI

Malawi counts as one of the poorest sub-Saharan countries, and the facts are grim: a GNI of US$280 per capita in 2009, more than half of the population living below the poverty line in 2009, and an average life expectancy of fifty-six years for men, fifty-seven for women. The Malawi government officially acknowledged widespread infection with HIV among its population only in 2004, but has since aimed to tackle the ensuing AIDS crisis by increasing funding for the health sector and for health education, both of which are starting to show some first effects (UNDP MDG 2010).[4] Only 17 per cent of Malawi's population lives in urban areas, with the remaining great majority living in rural areas, characterised at the best of times by difficulties in healthcare provision. Malawi's nurses and physicians, however, are concentrated in urban areas, with 25 per cent of them working at four urban health centres (WHO 2004). Child mortality rates, while in decline over recent years, are nevertheless still unconscionably high: in 2004, infant mortality was at 109 per 1,000 live births, the mortality for children under the age of five was recorded at 175 per 1,000 live births in the same year, with the biggest killers being neonatal causes, diarrhoea, malaria and pneumonia. For the period between 1990 and 2000, under-fives mortality rates in rural Malawi were determined at 210 deaths per 1,000 live births, compared to 148 deaths to 1,000 live births in urban areas. While the infant and under-fives mortality rates are in line with the average for the WHO African region, the maternal mortality rate in Malawi is high, with 1,800 mothers out of 100,000 having died in 2003 – nearly double the number of the WHO African comparison group (910). The mortality rate per 100,000 from HIV/AIDS is 681 in 2003, also more than double that of the comparison WHO African region (313) (all figures from WHO 2006). In fact, according to the WHO, the maternal mortality rate had increased dramatically between 1990, when it was at 560 per 100,000 per live births (and well below the WHO African region comparison of 860 for the same year) to 580 in 1995, after which it shot up to 1,800 per 100,000 live births in 2004. This suggests that maternal mortality and its increase are intimately linked to HIV/AIDS and its socio-economic consequences (Bicego et al. 2002). It also implies that lack of prevention and detection of HIV infection may be a contributing factor to the spread of the epidemic and the high death toll.

In an effort to improve health conditions among the population, the Malawi Health Department started a Health Initiative (with the help of NGOs and foreign aid) in 2004 to distribute healthcare packages aimed at addressing some of the most basic challenges to people's health, including test kits to determine HIV infection rates among women of birth age and pregnant women (Palmer 2006).[5] However, due to a lack of registered nurses in many rural areas, these kits were often administered by inexperienced healthcare assistants who often had received only ten weeks of training (Gondwe and Brysiewicz 2008). Registered nurses are the most valuable nurses since they are the most experienced. In order to provide incentives for registered nurses to stay in government services and not to move into either the private sector or abroad, the Malawi government has aimed to provide for better salaries and work conditions, particularly in rural areas where nurses have access to subsidised housing among other things – thus allowing for nurses to live a middle-class lifestyle (Palmer 2006).[6]

Most nurses in Malawi who emigrate choose to go to the UK – 317 did so between 2002 and 2005. In 2004, all of Malawi had access to 7,264 nurses, which translated to 0.59 nurses per 1,000 inhabitants,[7] with no midwives at all to report. Recall here the WHO's definition of undersupply as any number below 1.71 nurses per 1,000 inhabitants (WHO 2009: 15). In the same year, seventy-nine registered nurses were validated to move abroad, sixty-seven of whom went to the UK.[8] This is to say that in one year, nearly 1.5 per cent of registered nurses left Malawi for other shores (Palmer 2006: 31).

In the same year that the Malawi government implemented its health initiative in 2004, the UK government adopted the NHS Code for International Recruitment, which was meant to reduce international recruitment that would inflict harm on sending societies, thereby making immigration for Malawi nurses more difficult (Palmer 2006: 35).[9] Yet nurses continue to emigrate to the UK – certainly one reason for which is the much higher value their labour gains them there. Any salary increases the Malawi government can offer will never be able to compare – even in the more expensive context of the UK – with salaries accessible in developed countries (see Record and Mohidin 2006).

Based on the figures above, we can establish the kind of moral wrong that the emigration of Malawi nurses causes: we can safely say that

Malawians, particularly young children in rural areas and pregnant women, are more vulnerable to suffering from diseases than others due to a lack of access to early detection and preventative treatments. If they had access to a nurse, we can speculate that this would not have happened, that these same diseases might have been detected and successfully treated. We can also speculate that if Malawi nurses weren't able to emigrate or if emigration was very difficult and involved overcoming onerous restrictions, they might choose to remain in the country, potentially also moving to the countryside considering the kinds of advantages the government aims to provide them with if they do so. The link established between vulnerability and a moral wrong that I think necessary to justify exit restrictions, however, warrants exploration. In the following section, I explain why I posit that not protecting the vulnerable constitutes a moral wrong.

What Kind of Vulnerability?

'Vulnerability' can describe different things. A very general proposition is that vulnerability describes that part of our lives in which we are 'under threat of harm' (Goodin 1985: 110). The term may be employed to describe simple *background conditions* when thinking about persons and how they should be treated. To give quite an obvious example, the physical vulnerability of a newborn or a young child is a simple background condition of the life of a newborn or a child, even though we need not assume that most or even many children will be abused or neglected. The idea of human vulnerability then tries to account for human limitations and attempts to capture the 'fragility of human life, action and achievement' (O'Neill 1998).[10]

Bioethicists have tried to propose a more refined definition of human vulnerability as a background condition that aims to account for differences in vulnerability based on *likelihood* of harm and *ability* to protect oneself. For instance, we can imagine that we are all vulnerable to being attacked in the streets; but among an average population, we can identify some who are more vulnerable to be attacked than others – children, for instance, women and the very old, all of whom can easily be overwhelmed physically. However, it is of course not the case that all women are equally vulnerable or under the threat of harm. A second and very important component to a useful definition of vulnerability, then, needs to account for the ability to prevent the advent of harm.

In this instance, we could say that young children are always vulnerable everywhere, but that women may be very able to prevent harm to themselves. Finally, we need to consider whether harm is likely – whether, that is, a person finds herself in the situation in which her vulnerability will most likely lead to harm against which she will not be able to protect herself. Taking stock of what determines whether or not we are actually 'under the threat of harm', a useful concept of vulnerability may be to say that 'to be vulnerable means to face a significant probability of incurring an identifiable harm while substantially lacking ability and/or means to protect oneself' (Schroeder and Gefenas 2009: 117).

Vulnerability is not always morally problematic. Children and women may be described as being vulnerable, but the moral relevance doesn't derive from their being vulnerable since many would agree that we are all vulnerable in some way. To be vulnerable, in other words, is in the first instance an analysis of the state of the world, not a moral claim. The moral relevance argument has to be provided from somewhere else, namely that harm could have been prevented, but hasn't been prevented, for unjustified reasons.[11] The *moral* wrong inflicted in the case of Malawi, then, is not that many women and children fall ill and die but rather, that there are many accessible ways to prevent many of the diseases that lead to high mortality rates but that these preventative and therapeutic measures are not employed in the rural areas. Assessing the situation of healthcare provision in Malawi through the lens of vulnerability, then, I argue that the vulnerability of children and women of child-bearing age is undeniable – the lives of women and children in Malawi are characterised by a lack of effective protection against diseases due to a lack of detection, prevention and treatment. In fact, we may go as far as to say that a lack of prevention constitutes the ground for establishing 'a significant probability of incurring an identifiable harm', while lack of detection and treatment contributes to the 'substantial lack of means to protect oneself' against the harm that comes with the disease. The moral wrong that results from this, finally, is that such protection and treatment is available somewhere, but not in all of Malawi. Note here that the under-fives mortality rate in urban areas has historically been 25 per cent lower (148 per 1,000) than that of rural under-fives (210 per 1,000).[12]

Now, and in order to make a justice-based argument for exit restrictions for healthcare-workers in Malawi, a link needs to be made between the moral harm that results from background vulnerability in Malawi, and the emigration of healthcare professionals in Malawi. In other words, we need to ask if women and under-fives would be able to have access to prevention and treatment – to effective prevention against harm – if registered nurses were not to emigrate, but rather chose to stay in the country. The claim by those advocating exit restrictions, as far as I understand it, is that emigration of healthcare-workers puts into question the viability of the Malawi healthcare sector to the point of inflicting morally relevant vulnerability. The numbers recorded above documenting the implementation of Malawi's 2004 healthcare package seem to suggest that an increase in the number of health professionals is the remedy of choice for the Malawi government (see Palmer 2006; UNDP 2010), and granted that the retained nurses would actually work in the public sector and serve in rural areas, we can accept that this might be a way to address the problem of accessibility to prevention and treatment in rural areas. The argument from vulnerability, then, seems to support exit restrictions for Malawi nurses.

2. WHY MALAWI NURSES EMIGRATE: INDIVIDUAL AUTONOMY AND PERSONAL GOALS

How should we balance the realisation of goals Malawi nurses have set for themselves against the good of protecting against vulnerability of children and women in Malawi? I posit that justice considerations are contextual. This is to say that we may find that principles of justice that apply in one context don't actually promote justice in another context (see Carens 2004). From a principled-only perspective, we may be led to believe, in other words, that the emigration of Malawi nurses results in an injustice toward members of the society of origin, which trained them and enabled them to become nurses. Yet assessing the effects of exit restrictions in the specific case of Malawi's nurses, I posit, may show that the implementation of a principle-based exit restriction in fact challenges and potentially jeopardises another commensurable moral good, that of individual autonomy and self-determination. This is the claim of this section: that emigration can serve the moral goods of individual autonomy. In order to sustain this claim, I will provide a very brief account of the motivation for Malawi women to become nurses, and contextualise these choices with the opportunities open to them in Malawi compared to those open through emigration. I will argue that becoming a nurse and emigrating allows women to realise two moral goods: it provides them with autonomy-relevant opportunities, while also allowing them to provide for their families.

I endorse a definition of autonomy that relies on the idea of self-determination and self-realisation (see Meyers 2002). To be self-determining, individuals need to be able to set themselves goals and have a chance of realising these same goals. Self-determination as I construe it thus requires access to a range of viable options and opportunities (see Raz 1986). Many nurses provide different reasons for their entry into the profession – most common among younger nurses are reasons of financial security and the fact that the profession provides a way of earning a good salary, especially if employment is found with an international NGO or abroad (Grigulis et al. 2009). Nurses do well in Malawi society: the ratio between Malawi's GNI per person (US$800 in 2005) and nurses' GNI was 54 for nurses with international NGOs, and 36.5 for the nurses with local NGOs. And while these ratios were higher than those recorded for public-sector nurses (McCoy et al. 2008: 679), public-sector nurses were nevertheless provided with squarely middle-class incomes.[13] These figures, however, should be read critically since level of salary is not the best and only determinant of assessing how easily costs of living can be met (see McCoy et al. 2008: 677) or whether individual goals can be realised. And indeed, as many studies show, the salary level is not the sole determinant of job satisfaction; rather, this depends on a confluence of factors that are presented in different constellations, such as the workload, the equipment of hospitals, and the danger nurses perceive themselves to be in when carrying out their work, to name but the most important criteria (see Mangham and Hanson 2008; see also Brock 2009a). Working conditions are better in the UK than in Malawi. Leaving aside for the time being the differences in salary, nurses work in environments that are on average better equipped than those available in Malawi, under conditions that are less stressful – compare the stress of having to assist mothers in childbirth in the UK compared to Malawi, for instance, or the possibility of providing a cure to the sick in both countries.

Many nurses discussing job satisfaction not only mention salary levels and working conditions, but also better opportunities for family members, for example in the form of good schools and providing further opportunities for children. Such goals are a driving push factor for emigration (McCoy et al. 2008: 680; see also Kingsma 2006: Chapter

1). We can assume that many nurses are motivated to emigrate by the idea of providing opportunities for family members through the fruits of their work; a variable that takes on prominence if they find themselves to be the sole breadwinner in the family. This part of individual autonomy is important, it seems to me, since it denotes a motivation that is not simply individualistic but extends to the duties women nurses feel they have for the welfare of those closest to them.

What is the evidence for this to be successful? Particularly, how does emigration affect the welfare of family members left behind? This is difficult to assess since figures for remittance payments as an indicator of realising the goal of taking care of families are hard to find for Malawi. Until such figures are available, approximations will have to do. A survey including different nationalities of foreign recruited nurses in London states that most foreign nurses 'reported they were the major or sole wage-earner contributing to household income. More than half of the respondents (57%) reported that they regularly sent remittances to their home country' (Buchan et al. 2006: 1481).[14] This is in line with figures gathered for nurses as a migratory labour force, which has contributed $100 billion worldwide in remittances in 2004 alone (Keith 2007: 356). Women nurses thus choose emigration to realise some important responsibilities toward family members at home.[15]

Recall, however, that figures given earlier suggest that Malawi nurses have many options to provide for families also if they stay in Malawi – especially considering their standard of living in comparison to other Malawians. One way of addressing the challenge of balancing the vulnerability of mothers and children in rural Malawi compared to the realisation of individual goals of Malawi nurses might thus be to search for a definition of what exactly viable options are. This choice of argument, however, is based on a concept of the realm of options that is clearly no longer accepted by high-skilled workers around the globe, and furthermore not obviously defendable from a moral perspective. Put differently, it is not clear why we should accept the boundaries of the national community only as the measure for comparison of what counts as viable options. As many cosmopolitan egalitarians have argued, and as the movement of nurses and other foreign workers around the globe attests, the measure of comparison for those with skills in demand are options anywhere, especially in countries that are willing to hire them – not only those available in the country of origin. I refer here to the premise of moral cosmopolitanism that stipulates that the moral equality of human beings requires the extension of measures of justice beyond the realm of the nation-state. When assessing the conditions of individual autonomy, then, it can't simply be assumed that the opportunities available in the country of origin only should determine our moral assessment of these conditions. Instead, I argue that opportunities for nurses everywhere need to be taken into account when determining what individual autonomy for them implies.[16]

Note also that those proposing exit restrictions on healthcare-workers will accept this framework of analysis: the motivation underlying concern about brain drain, it seems to me, is a concern for global justice or, at least, a concern about the effects of fundamental global *in*justice. Theorists who worry about brain drain plausibly do so because they worry about conditions of life in one country compared to those in another. If that is the case, however, then such arguments are based on a cosmopolitan premise, which is to say that we care, to some extent, for the well-being of individuals everywhere.

3. EXIT RESTRICTIONS AND MORAL GOODS

So far, I have accepted that emigration of nurses may be accepted to cause a moral wrong for at least two sub-sections of Malawi society – rural mothers and under-5-year-olds. I have also accepted that this wrong is a consequence of vulnerability as a background condition of their lives, due to a lack of prevention and treatment. I have also accepted that if more nurses were available, we can speculate that more prevention and treatment could be administered. I have then proposed that from a contextual stance, this is not enough to justify exit restrictions, since such restrictions need to pass the proportionality test: those proposing restrictions need to show that no comparable and commensurable good is challenged or jeopardised through such restrictions.[17] The good I have juxtaposed to the protections against vulnerability is that of individual autonomy. I have argued that for nurses to be autonomous they need to be able to realise important goals in their life. Two such goals are to work in rewarding circumstances, and to provide for opportunities for family members. I have posited these two moral goods – protection against harm due to vulnerability *and* the realisation of individual autonomy – as commensurable. In this section, I want to argue that some exit restrictions may be justifiable; however, the form they would need to take in order *not* to jeopardise the second moral good of individual autonomy might make them an ineffective tool of global justice.

I consider two kinds of exit restrictions: an exit tax, and imposed service after the end of training. We could propose that trained nurses should be required to serve for five years in the country of training, say. Such a restriction, however, violates the realisation of individual goals, and doesn't simply delay them temporarily, as one might think. Imagine the case of a young nurse recently graduated who has decided to emigrate in order to provide for the education of her brother. A delay in her emigration, however, would not allow her to realise this goal since five years down the road, the brother would be too old or would have had to take on a job. Now, to be sure, we could say that we face restrictions in our realisation of goals frequently, and often they have to do with monetary need. However, the restriction here would not be based on the personal circumstances of the nurse, or her brother, but simply on the fact that society imposes duties on her toward its members that supposedly supersede those she has adopted and accepted toward her family members. This seems like a harmless case, but imagine the same nurse to have a mother who is ill with cancer – a disease for which she could receive treatment, but only if she were to travel to South Africa and stay there for the duration of the treatment, say. Her health access in a foreign country would not be covered by her Malawi national health plan, and so would depend on her own financial resources. Here we could say that a delay in allowing her daughter to emigrate in order to earn the funds would impose an unproportional burden on her, for the benefit of the healthcare system of the country. This would not be a morally neutral measure since it would not allow the nurse to fulfil her duties of care toward her mother.

A more promising venue would be to impose an exit tax on those who aim to emigrate. The tax would still allow the nurse to emigrate and to fulfil her duties toward her family members, while also paying some amount back to the sending community. However, such a tax would have to be quite small in amount if it were meant to be morally neutral: in order for nurses still to be able to realise their individual goals (by sending money home, say) and taking into account the expenses of travel, and living in a foreign country, we could imagine that such a tax could only amount to a rather minimal sum. In particular, and keeping both goals in view, we could imagine that a tax should not be so high as to make nurses decide to stay longer in the host society, rather than return – a move a majority of them plan to make after a set period of time – since if they stayed longer their absence would harm the sending society further. It could also not be so high as to discourage young people from choosing nursing as a profession altogether, since this would be detrimental to the overall goal. We can then conclude that an exit tax proportional to the level of income and expense, and taking into account monies sent to the family back home, could be morally justifiable. Yet we may wonder what good such a restriction would be since a minimal tax would not likely discourage emigration and certainly not compensate for the loss of a valuable nurse. So while morally justifiable, and contextually adequate, we may wonder if such an exit tax would yield the desired outcome, which is to prevent moral wrong due to vulnerability to death from preventable diseases. Would it actually allow Malawi to train more nurses, or retain more of those trained?

A more straightforward measure (and one less plagued by moral hazards) is to shift the burden onto recruiting countries and to require them to pay a 'head tax' to sending countries. This could come in the form of direct compensation when providing for a nurse's visa, or as a contribution to further training facilities and the like (see Kapur and McHale 2006). There are good moral reasons for accepting such a head tax – the same reasons, in fact, that seem to have motivated the NHS to adopt its voluntary ethical recruitment guidelines. But, to be sure, some could argue that this would negate the advantage of recruiting countries: why should they then recruit from developing countries if the financial advantage diminishes? This is important for the moral balancing I am engaged in: if the UK decided to halt recruitment from Malawi, this would have fundamental effects on the individual's possibility to seek opportunities elsewhere. In other words, if recruiting countries stopped processing visas from countries of origin, might my proposal not jeopardise one of the two moral goods I aim to protect, namely to provide opportunities to individuals?

Recall here the numbers provided earlier: the costs to train a doctor in the UK, even if we only take the lowest level of training, still amount to at least five times the costs of a doctor's training in the country of origin. Put differently, even if the UK compensated Kenya for the entire costs of training a doctor accumulated between primary school and graduation from medical school, the overall gain would still be very high for the UK. It is not clear, then, that the UK or any other country recruiting from developing countries would stop doing so when obliged to pay its fair share of education costs, instead of free-riding on the education paid for by developing sending societies.

CONCLUSION

Healthcare professionals moving from healthcare-poor countries to healthcare-rich countries leads to a lack of access to healthcare. This in turn provokes situations in which background conditions of vulnerability to be infected and to die of preventable diseases turns into a moral wrong that could be averted if more healthcare professionals were spread evenly across the country. However, to lay the burden on the individual who aims to emigrate doesn't seem to be a defendable solution to the problem of brain drain, since the competing moral good of individual autonomy is jeopardised if we restrict the opportunities people have to realise their migration project. Instead, the brain drain should be considered a problem of global redistributive justice, with those countries benefiting from recruitment of foreign-trained healthcare-workers under an obligation to compensate the countries that trained them.

Notes

1. This is not a definition that effectively evaluates how well individuals will be able to live and I don't aim to propose such a definition here. For discussion of some such measures, see the chapters by Asada, Venkatapuram and Voigt in this volume.
2. Note that the losses in returns for the training country's investment are estimated to be nearly eight times the cost for training the individual healthcare practitioner (Kirigia et al. 2006).
3. The pernicious consequences of skilled outmigration go beyond losing valuable professionals: because public finances of sending countries deteriorate due to the loss in investment return, some countries then can't actually employ the health professionals that are in the country for lack of funds (see WHO 2009).
4. According to the Malawi government, the percentage of pregnant women (aged 15–24 years) infected with HIV, for instance, has decreased from 24.1 per cent in 1998 to 12 per cent in 2009 (UNDP MDG 2010: 38)
5. The dangers arising from the combination of being a woman and living in a country where AIDS is so widespread is underlined by Palmer: 'In 2004,

out of 540,000 deliveries only 7.9% women were tested for HIV. A meagre 2.7% of pregnant women in need of ARV prophylaxis received the intervention' (Palmer 2006: 31).

6. See Gorman (2009), in which she records her findings from interviews she conducted in her position as a Fellow at Harvard's School of Public Health and the accompanying photo-essay by her travel companion Eileen Hohmuth-Lemonick (2011).

7. To complete this picture, Palmer reports 1.1 physicians on 100,000 inhabitants for 2003 (Palmer 2006: 29)

8. Overall, between 2000 and 2011, only 684 registered nurses have graduated in Malawi (email communication from Martha Mondiwa, Nurses and Midwife Council of Malawi, 10 November 2011).

9. However, some argue that these measures have not actually prevented outmigration, but since implemented voluntarily, have either not changed the migration patterns much or have driven nurses into illegality (Migration Watch 2004).

10. I distinguish vulnerability as a *background condition of one's life*, which may warrant special attention and care, from the specific vulnerability that is the result of somebody's actions, what I will call *induced vulnerability*. The vulnerability of one person in this sense may directly result from the actions of another agent. This second kind of vulnerability always causes moral wrong when it results in harm to another because of the accepted moral obligation to take responsibility for those of our actions that harm others. I don't think the case for this kind of vulnerability can be made in Malawi since it ascribes individual responsibility to individual nurses, and so I will neglect it here. For a treatment of responsibility, see Brock and Haussman, this volume.

11. The 'unjustified' clause is important here: we can imagine a situation of resource scarcity, in which a government has to decide how to spend its (meagre) resources. Assume that children need access to malaria nets (which are inexpensive to provide and very effective if applied properly) but that the society in question has suffered a drought and needs to first and foremost spend its resources on food imports to avert a famine. Under such a scenario, we could accept that a lack of prevention of malaria can be justified, even if we may wish that prevention was kept in place.

12. The measure of justice here is a luck egalitarian one that posits (very simply put) that it is unjust to die of these diseases for the bad luck of living in a rural area with lack of access to health provision, while some others share the good luck of living close to urban healthcare centres that can provide access (see Segall 2010).

13. This position is often buttressed by searching for the best bundle of 'allowances': these include such special payments for food, clothing and

housing, often employed to attract health professionals to accept positions in rural areas.

14. It is noteworthy here that most of the nurses of the survey (60 per cent) were 40 years or older, married and with children.

15. This is not to say, of course, that some of the expectations migrant nurses have may not be fulfilled (see Kingsma 2006: Chapter 1).

16. This is not to say that a viable range of options in my definition of autonomy requires the need to *maximise* options. I don't accept that individuals have to have access to the best or the most options in order to be autonomous. This doesn't imply, however, that their options can simply be circumscribed by national boundaries.

17. Note that from a different perspective, one could argue that any justification of exit restrictions would also have to show that the individual restricted is the one best capable of protecting against vulnerability, rather than somebody else. I will not pursue this argument here, but see Oberman (2011).

BIBLIOGRAPHY

Ahmed, K., Smith, J. and Whiteside, A. (2009). 'Global Funding of the AIDS Response'. *Newsletter of the International AIDS Society*, 8–9.

Alkire, S. and Chen, L. (2006). '"Medical Exceptionalism" in International Migration: Should Doctors and Nurses be Treated Differently?' In K. Tamas and J. Palma, (eds), *Globalizing Migration Regimes: New Challenges to Transnational Cooperation*. Aldershot: Ashgate.

Allotey, P., Reidpath, D., Kouamé, A. and Cummins, R. (2003). 'The DALY, Ccntext and the Determinants of the Severity of Disease: An Exploratory Comparison of Paraplegia in Australia and Cameroon'. *Social Science and Medicine*, 57(5), 949–58.

Anand, S. and Hanson, K. (1997). 'Disability-adjusted Life Years: A Critical Review'. *Journal of Health Economics*, 16(6), 685–702.

Anand, S. (2002). 'The Concern for Equity in Health'. *Journal of Epidemiology and Community Health*, 56, 485–87.

Anderson, E. (1999). 'What is the Point of Equality?' *Ethics*, 109 (January), 287–337.

Anderson, E. (2010). 'Justifying the Capabilities Approach to Justice'. In H. Brighouse and I. Robeyns (eds), *Measuring Justice. Primary Goods and Capabilities*. Cambridge: Cambridge University Press.

Anderson, M. B. (1998). 'You Save My Life Today, But for What Tomorrow? Some Moral Dilemmas of Humanitarian Aid'. In J. Moore (ed.), *Hard Choices: Moral Dilemmas in Humanitarian Intervention* (Vol. 137–156). Lanham, MD: Rowman and Littlefield.

Angell, M. (2004). *The Truth About the Drug Companies: How They Deceive Us and What To Do About It*. New York: Random House.

Arnesen, T. and Kapiriri, L. (2004). 'Can the Value Choices in DALYs Influence Global Priority-Setting?' *Health Policy*, 70(2), 137–149.

Arnesen, T. and Nord, E. (1999). The Value of DALY Life: Problems with Ethics and Validity of Disability Adjusted Life Years'. *British Medical Journal*, 319, 1423–5.

265

Arneson, R. (1989). 'Equality and Equal Opportunity for Welfare'. *Philosophical Studies*, 56, 77–93.

Asada, Y. and Hedermann, T. (2002). 'A Problem with the Individual Approach in the WHO Health Inequality Measurement'. *International Journal for Equity in Health*, 1(2), 1–5.

Asada, Y. (2005). 'Medical Technologies, Nonhuman Aids, Human Assistance, and Environmental Factors in the Assessment of Health States'. *Quality of Life Research*, 14(3), 867–74.

Asada, Y. (2007). *Health Inequality: Morality and Measurement*. Toronto: University of Toronto Press.

Bach, S. (2003). *Migration of Health Workers: Labour and Social Issues*. Geneva: ILO.

Baker, R. (2005). *Capitalism's Achilles Heel: Dirty Money and How to Renew the Free-Market System*. Hoboken, NJ: John Wiley & Sons.

Barnett, M. (2005). 'Humanitarianism Transformed'. *Perspectives on Politics*, 3(4), 723–40.

Barry, B. (1998). 'International Society from a Cosmopolitan Perspective'. In D. Maple and T. Nardin (eds), *International Society: Diverse Ethical Perspectives* (pp. 144–61). New Jersey: Princeton University Press.

Barry, C. and G. Overland (2010). 'Why Remittances to the Poor Should Not be Taxed'. *Journal of International Politics and Law*, 42, 1181–207.

Barry, C. (2011). 'Immigration and Global Justice'. *Global Justice: Theory Practice Rhetoric*, 4.

Beck, U. (2006). *Cosmopolitan Vision*. Cambridge Polity Press.

Beitz, C. (1979). 'Justice and International Relations'. *Philosophy and Public Affairs*, 4(4), 360–89.

Beitz, C. (1992). 'International Liberalism and Distributive Justice: A Survey of Recent Thought'. *World Politics*, 52(1), 269–96.

Beitz, C. (2009). *The Idea of Human Rights*. Oxford: Oxford University Press.

Bell, D. A. and Carens, J. H. (2004). 'The Ethical Dilemmas of International Human Rights and Humanitarian NGOs: Reflections on a Dialogue between Practitioners and Theorists'. *Human Rights Quarterly*, 26(2), 300–29.

Benatar, S. and Upshur, R. (2011). 'What is Global Health?' In S. Benatar and G. Brock (eds), *Global Health and Global Health Ethics* (pp. 14–15). Cambridge: Cambridge University Press.

Bergson, H. (1911). *Creative Evolution* (A. Mitchell, trans.). New York: Henry Holt.

Berkman, L. F. and Kawachi, I. O. (2000). *Social Epidemiology*. New York: Oxford University Press.

Berliner, H. S. and Ginzberg, E. (2002). 'Why this Hospital Nursing Shortage is Different'. *Journal of the American Medical Association*, 288, 2742–4.

BIO Ventures for Global Health. (2011). 'Priority Review Vouchers', from http://www.bvgh.org/What-We-Do/Incentives/Priority-Review-Vouchers. aspx

Birn, A.-E. (2011). 'Addressing the Societal Determinants of Health'. In S. Benatar and G. Brock (eds), *Global Health and Global Health Ethics* (pp. 37–53). Cambridge: Cambridge University Press.

Bognar, G. (2008). 'Age-weighting'. *Economics and Philosophy*, 24(2), 167–89.

Boorse, C. (1977). 'Health as a Theoretical Concept'. *Philosophy of Science*, 44, 542–73.

Boorse, C. (1997). 'A Rebuttal on Health'. In R. Almeder (ed.), *What Is Disease?* (Vol. 1–134). Totowa, NJ: Humana Press.

Booth, K. (2007). *Theory of World Security*. Cambridge: Cambridge University Press.

Brasil Ministerio de Salud (2011). *Tabela de Preços*. Retrieved from http://portal. saude.gov.br/portal/arquivos/pdf/tabela_farmaciapopular_abril08.pdf

Braveman, P., Krieger, N. and Lynch, J. (2000). 'Health Inequalities and Social Inequalities in Health'. *Bulletin of the World Health Organization*, 78(2), 232–3.

Braveman, P., Starfield, B., Geiger, H. J. and Murray, C. J. L. (2001). 'World Health Report 2000: How it Removes Equity from the Agenda for Public Health Monitoring and Policy'. *Bulletin of the World Health Organization*, 323, 678–81.

Braveman, P. and Gruskin, S. (2003). 'Defining Equity in Health'. *Journal of Epidemiology and Community Health*, 57(4), 254–8.

Braveman, P. (2006). 'Health Disparities and Health Equity: Concepts and Measurement'. *Annual Review of Public Health*, 27, 167–94.

Brock, D. (2002). 'The Separability of Health and Well-being'. In C. Murray, J. Salomon, C. Mathers and A. Lopez (eds), *Summary of Measures of Population Health: Ethics, Measurement and Applications* (Vol. 115–120). Geneva: WHO.

Brock, G. (2005). 'Needs and Global Justice'. In S. Reader (ed.), *The Philosophy of Need* (pp. 51–72). Cambridge: Cambridge University Press.

Brock, G. (2008). 'Taxation and Global Justice: Closing the Gap between Theory and Practice'. *Journal of Social Philosophy*, 39(2), 161–84.

Brock, G. (2009a). 'Health in Developing Countries and Our Global Responsibilities'. In A. Dawson (ed.), *The Philosophy of Public Health* (pp. 73–90). Aldershot: Ashgate.

Brock, G. (2009b). *Global Justice: A Cosmopolitan Account*. Oxford: Oxford University Press.

Broome, J. (2002). 'Measuring the Burden of Disease by Aggregating Well-being'. In C. Murray, J. Salomon, C. Mathers and A. Lopez (eds), *Summary Measures of Population Health: Concepts, Ethics, Measurement and Applications* (Vol. 91–113). Geneva: WHO.

Broome, J. (2005). 'Should We Value Population?' *The Journal of Political Philosophy*, 13(4), 399–413.

Brown, G. W. and Labonte, R. (2011). 'Globalization and its Methodological Discontents: Contextualizing Globalization Through the Study of HIV/AIDS'. *Globalization and Health*, 7(29).

Buchan, J., Parkin, T. and Sochalski, J. (2003). *International Nurse Mobility: Trends and Policy Implications*. Geneva: WHO.

Buchan, J., Jobanputra, R., Gough, P. and Hutt, R. (2006). 'Internationally Recruited Nurses in London: A Survey of Career Paths and Plans'. *Human Resources for Health*, 4(14), 1478–91.

Buchanan, A. (1984). 'The Right to a Decent Minimum of Health Care'. *Philosophy and Public Affairs*, 13(1), 55–78.

Buchanan, A., Brock, D., Daniels, N. and Wikler, D. (2000). *From Change to Choice: Genetics and Justice*. Cambridge: Cambridge University Press.

Buchanan, A. (2009). *Justice and Health Care: Selected Essays*. Oxford: Oxford University Press.

Buchanan, A. and DeCamp, M. (2011). 'Responsibility for Global Health'. In S. Benatar and G. Brock (eds), *Global Health and Global Health Ethics* (pp. 119–28). Cambridge: Cambridge University Press.

Buchanan-Smith, M. and Fabbri, P. (2005). *Linking Relief, Rehabilitation and Development – A Review of the Debate*. Tsunami Evaluation Coalition.

Bunnell, R., Mermin, J. and Cock, K. M. d. (2006). 'HIV Prevention for a Threatened Continent: Implementing Positive Prevention in Africa'. *Journal of the American Medical Association*, 297(7), 855–8.

Cabrera, L. (2010). *The Practice of Global Citizenship*. Cambridge: Cambridge University Press.

Caney, S. (2005). *Justice Beyond Borders: A Global Political Theory*. Oxford: Oxford University Press.

Caney, S. (2011). 'Humanity, Associations and Global Justice: In Defense of Humanity-centred Egalitarianism'. *The Monist*, 94(4).

Carens, J. (2004). 'A Contextual Approach to Political Theory'. *Ethical Theory and Moral Practice*, 7(2), 117–32.

Casey, E. S. (1997). *The Fate of Place: A Philosophical History*. Berkeley: University of California Press.

Casey, E. S. (1999). 'The Tie of the Glance: Toward Becoming Otherwise'. In E. Grosz (ed.), *Becomings: Explorations in Time, Memory, and Futures*. Ithaca, NY: Cornell University Press.

Chatterji, S., Üstün, B., Sadana, R., Salomon, J., Mathers, C. and Murray, C. (2002). 'The Conceptual Basis for Measuring and Reporting Health'. *Global Programme on Evidence for Health Policy Discussion Paper*.

Code, L. (2006). *Ecological Knowing: The Politics of Epistemic Location*. Oxford: Oxford University Press.

'Code of Conduct for The International Red Cross and Red Crescent Movement and NGOs in Disaster Relief' (2003). *World Disasters Report 2003: Focus on ethics in aid*. Geneva: IFRC.

Cohen, G. A. (1989). 'On the Currency of Egalitarian Justice'. *Ethics*, 89, 906–44.

Cole, P. (1998). *The Free, the Unfree and the Excluded: A Treatise on the Conditions of Liberty*. Aldershot: Ashgate.

Cole, P. (2007). 'Human Rights and the National Interest: Migrants, Health Care and Social Justice'. *Journal of Medical Ethics*, 33(5), 269–72.

Cole, P. (2009). 'Migration and the Human Right to Health'. *Cambridge Quarterly of Health Care Ethics*, 19(1), 70–7.

Connel, J. (2010). *Migration and the Globalization of Health Care: The Health Worker Exodus?* Northampton, MA: Edward Elgar Publishing.

Connell, J. and Stilwell, B. (2006). 'Recruiting Agencies in the Global Health Care Chain'. In C. Kuptsch (ed.), *Merchants of Labour*. Geneva: International Labour Organization.

Cooper, E. R., Charurat, M., Mofenson, L., Hanson, C., Pitt, J., Diaz, C. and Blattner, W. (2002). 'Combination Antiretroviral Strategies for the Treatment of Pregnant HIV-1-infected Women and Prevention of Perinatal HIV-1 Transmission'. *Journal of Acquired Immune Deficiency Syndromes*, 29(5), 484–94.

Cranston, M. (1983). 'Are There Any Human Rights?' *Daedalus*, 112 (Fall).

Crawley, H. (2010). 'Chance or Choice? Understanding why Asylum Seekers Come to the UK', at: http://www.refugeecouncil.org.uk/policy/briefings/2010/13012010_x

Creese, A., Floyd, K., Alban, A. and Guinness, L. (2002). 'Cost-effectiveness of HIV/AIDS Interventions in Africa: A Systematic Review of the Evidence'. [Review]. *Lancet*, 359 (9318), 1635–43.

Culp, J. and Hassoun, N. (2011). 'Bridging the Gap in Scientific Research'. In D. Scott (ed.), *Debating Science: Deliberation, Values and the Common Good*. Amherst: Prometheus.

Daniels, N. (1981). 'Health-care Needs and Distributive Justice'. *Philosophy & Public Affairs*, 10(2), 146–79.

Daniels, N. (1985). *Just Health Care*. Cambridge: Cambridge University Press.

Daniels, N. (2007). 'Rescuing Universal Health Care'. *Hastings Center Report*, 37(2).

Daniels, N. (2008). *Just Health: Meeting Health Needs Fairly*. Cambridge: Cambridge University Press.

Daniels, N. (2011). 'International Health Inequalities and Global Justice: Toward a Middle Ground'. In S. Benatar and G. Brock (eds), *Global Health and Global Health Ethics* (pp. 97–107). Cambridge: Cambridge University Press.

Davies, S. (2010). *Global Politics of Health*. Cambridge: Polity Press.

Deaton, A. (2003). 'Health, Inequality, and Economic Development'. *Journal of Economic Literature*, 41, 113–58.

Department of Health (2010). *Review of Access to the NHS by Foreign Nationals*. London: Crown.

Desgrees-Du-Lou, A., Msellati, P., Viho, I., Yao, A., Yapi, D., Kassi, P. and Dabis, F. (2002). 'Contraceptive Use, Protected Sexual Intercourse and Incidence of Pregnancies among African HIV-Infected Women'. DITRAME ANRS 049 Project, Abidjan 1995–2000. *International Journal of STD AIDS*, 13(7), 462–8.

Diaz, J. (2011). 'Apocalypse. What Disasters Reveal'. *Boston Review* (May/June).

Donagan, A. (1977). *Theory of Common Morality*. University of Chicago Press.

Dovlo, D. (2007). 'Migration of Nurses from Sub-Saharan Africa'. *Health Services Research*, 42(3), 1373–88.

Doyal, L. and Payne, S. (2011). 'Gender and Global Health: Inequality and Differences'. In S. Benatar and G. Brock (eds), *Global Health and Global Health Ethics* (pp. 53–62). Cambridge: Cambridge University Press.

Drummond, M. (2001). 'Introducing Economic and Quality of Life Measurements into Clinical Studies. *Annals of Medicine*, 22(5), 344–9.

Dworkin, R. (1981). 'What is Equality? Part 2: Equality of Resources'. *Philosophy and Public Affairs*, 10, 283–345.

Dworkin, R. (2000). *Sovereign Virtue*. Cambridge, MA: Harvard University Press.

Embrey, M., Hoos, D. and Quick, J. (2009). 'How AIDS Funding Strengthens Health Systems: Progress in Pharmaceutical Management'. *Journal of Acquired Immune Deficiency Syndromes*, 52 Suppl 1, S34-37.

Enarson, E. and Dhar Chakrabarti, P. G. (2009). *Women, Gender and Disaster: Global Issues and Initiatives*. Los Angeles: Sage.

Enarson, E. F. A. and Peek, L. (2006). 'Gender and Disaster: Foundations and Possibilities'. In H. Rodriguez, E. L. Quarantelli and R. Dynes (eds), *Handbook of Disaster Research* (Vol. 130–146). New York: Springer.

Evans, R. G. and Stoddart, G. L. (1990). 'Producing Health, Consuming Health Care'. *Social Science and Medicine*, 31, 1347–63.

Evans, T., Whitehead, M., Diderichsen, F., Bhuiya, A. and Wirth, M. (2001). *Challenging Inequities in Health: From Ethics to Action*. Oxford and New York: Oxford University Press.

Ezzati, M., Vander Hoorn, S., Lopez, A., Danaei, G., Rodgers, A., Mathers, C. et al. (2006). 'Comparative Quantification of Mortality and Burden of Disease Attributable to Selected Risk Factors'. In A. Lopez, C. Mathers, M. Ezzati and D. Jamison (eds), *Global Burden of Disease and Risk Factors* (2nd edn, pp. 241–68). Washington, DC: The World Bank and Oxford University Press.

Fairchild, A. L. and Oppenheimer, G. M. (1998). 'Public Health Nihilism vs

Pragmatism: History, Politics, and the Control of Tuberculosis'. *American Journal of Public Health*, 88(7), 1105–17.

Farmer, P. (2005). *Pathologies of Power. Health, Human Rights, and the New War on the Poor*. Berkeley: University of California Press.

Farmer, P. (2011a). *How to Rebuild Haiti after the Quake*. Paper presented at the Expert Roundup, Council on Foreign Relations.

Farmer, P. (2011b). *Haiti after the Earthquake*. New York: Perseus Books Group.

Fidler, D. (1999). *International Law and Infectious Diseases*. Oxford: Clarendon Press.

Fleurbaey, M. and Schokkaert, E. (2009). 'Unfair Inequalities in Health and Health Care'. *Journal of Health Economics*, 28(1), 73–90.

Flory, J. and Kitcher, P. (2004). 'Global Health and the Scientific Research Agenda'. *Philosophy and Public Affairs*, 32(1).

'Food and Drug Administration' (2008). OOPD Program Overview, from http://www.fda.gov/orphan/progovw.htm

Freeman, S. (2007). 'Rawls and Luck Egalitarianism'. In Freeman, S., *Justice and the Social Contract* (pp. 111–42). New York: Oxford University Press.

Furlong, W., Feeny, D., Torrance, G. W., Goldsmith, C. H., DePauw, S., Zhu. Z., Denton, M. and Boyle, M. (1998). 'Multiplicative Multi-attribute Utility Function for the HUI Mark 3 (HUI3) System: A Technical Report'. *CHEPA Working Paper Series*, 98(11).

Gakidou, E., Murray, C. J. L. and Frenk, J. (2000). 'A Framework for Measuring Health Inequality'. *Bulletin of the World Health Organization*, 78, 42–54.

Garrett, L. (2001). *Betrayal of Trust: The Collapse of Global Public Health*. Oxford: Oxford University Press.

Gill, S. and Bakker, I. (2011). 'The Global Crisis and Global Health'. In S. Benatar and G. Brock (eds), *Global Health and Global Health Ethics* (pp. 221–38). Cambridge: Cambridge University Press.

Global Health Workforce Alliance (2008). *The Kampala Declaration and Agenda for Global Action*. Paper presented at the First Global Forum on Human Resources for Health, Kampala, Uganda. http://www.who.int/workforceal-liance/ forum/2_declaration_final.pdf

Gondwe, W. D. M. and Brysiewicz, P. (2008). 'Emergency Nursing Experience in Malawi'. *International Emergency Nursing*, 16, 59–64.

Goodin, R. (1985). *Protecting the Vulnerable: A Re-analysis of our Social Responsibilities*. Chicago: Chicago University Press.

Goodin, R. (1998). 'Vulnerabilities and Responsibilities: An Ethical Defense of the Welfare State'. In G. Brock (ed.), *Necessary Goods: Our Responsibilities to Meet Others' Needs* (pp. 73–94). Oxford: Rowman and Littlefield.

Gostin, L. O. (2007). 'Why Rich Countries Should Care about the World's Least Healthy People'. *Journal of the American Medical Association*, 298(1), 89–92.

Gould, C. C. (2007a). 'Recognition, Empathy, and Solidarity'. In G. W. Bertram, R. Celikates, C. Laudou and D. Lauer (eds), *Socialite et Reconnaissance: Grammaires de l'Humain*. Paris: Editions L'Harmattan.

Gould, C. C. (2007b). 'Transnational Solidarities'. *Journal of Social Philosophy*, 38(1), 148–64.

Gould, C. C. (2009). 'Reconceiving Autonomy and Universality as Norms for Transnational Democracy'. In A. Langlois and K. Soltan (eds), *Global Democracy and Its Difficulties*. London: Routledge.

Graham, H. (2010). 'Where is the Future in Public Health?' *Milbank Quarterly*, 88(2), 149–68.

Griffin, J. (2002). 'A Note on Measuring Well-being.' *Summary Measures of Population Health: Concepts, Ethics, Measurement and Applications*. Geneva: WHO.

Griffin, J. (2008). *On Human Rights*. Oxford: Oxford University Press.

Grigulis, A. I., Post, A. and Osrin, D. (2009). 'The Lives of Malawian Nurses: The Stories Behind the Statistics'. *Transactions of the Royal Society of Tropical Medicine and Hygiene*, 103 (1195–6).

Grootendorst, P., Feeny, D. and Furlong, W. (2000). 'Health Utilities Index Mark 3 Evidence of Construct Validity for Stroke and Arthritis in a Population Health Survey'. *Medical Care*, 38(3), 290–9.

Grosz, E. (1995). 'Bodies-cities'. In E. Grosz (ed.), *Space, Time, and Perversion: Essays on the Politics of Bodies*. New York: Routledge.

Grosz, E. (1999). 'Thinking the New: Of Futures Yet Unthought'. In E. Grosz (ed.), *Becomings: Explorations in Time, Memory, and Futures*. Ithaca, NY: Cornell University Press.

'Growth of Aid and the Decline of Humanitarianism' (2010). *Lancet*, 375.

Hall, J. A. (1988). *Liberalism*. London: Paladin.

Hardin, G. (1968). 'The Tragedy of the Commons'. *Science*, 162(3859), 1243–8.

Hardin, G. (1974a). 'Lifeboat Ethics: The Case Against Helping the Poor'. *Psychology Today*, September.

Hardin, G. (1974b). 'Living on a Lifeboat'. *Bioscience*, 24(10), 561–8.

Harper, S. and Lynch, J. (2005). 'Methods for Measuring Cancer Disparities: Using Data Relevant to Healthy People 2010 Cancer-related Objectives'. *National Cancer Institute Cancer Surveillance Monograph Series*. Bethesda, MD: National Cancer Institute.

Harper, S., Lynch, J. and Smith, D. G. (2007). 'Trends in the Black–White life expectancy gap in the United States'. *Journal of the American Medical Association*, 297(11), 1224–32.

Hart, H. L. A. (1984). 'Are There Any Natural Rights?' In J. Waldron (ed.), *Theories of Rights*. Oxford: Oxford University Press.

Harvey, P. and Lind, J. (2005). *Dependency and Humanitarian Relief: A Critical Analysis*. London: Overseas Development Institute.

Hassoun, N. (forthcoming (a)). *Globalization and Global Justice: Shrinking Distance, Expanding Obligations.* Cambridge: Cambridge University Press.

Hassoun, N. (forthcoming (b)). 'Global Health Impact: A Basis for Labeling and Licensing Campaigns?' *Developing World Bioethics.*

Hausman, D. and McPherson, M. S. (2006). *Economic Analysis, Moral Philosophy and Public Policy* (2nd edition). New York: Cambridge University Press.

Hausman, D. (2006). 'Valuing Health'. *Philosophy and Public Affairs*, 34(3).

Hausman, D. (2007). 'Are Health Inequalities Unjust?' *Journal of Political Philosophy*, 15.

Hausman, D. (2009). 'Benevolence, Justice, Well-being and the Health Gradient'. *Public Health Ethics*, 2(3), 235–43.

Hausman, D. and Waldren M. S. (2011). 'Egalitarianism Reconsidered'. *Journal of Moral Philosophy*, 8, 1–20.

Hausman, D. (unpublished). *Summary Measures of Population Health: Some Conceptual Problems.*

Hay, S., Smith, D. and Snow, R. (2008). 'Measuring Malaria Endemicity from Intense to Interrupted Transmission'. *Lancet Infectious Diseases*, 8(6), 369–78.

Hay, S. (2009). 'A World Malaria Map: Plasmodium Falciparum Endemicity in 2007'. *PlosMedicine*, 286–302.

Health For All (2011). 'Smuggling is a Right: An open letter to the Canadian Council for Refugees on behalf of Health for All'. At: http://www.health4all.ca/node/32

'Health Tourism' rules unveiled (2003). *BBC News Online.* Retrieved from: http://news.bbc.co.uk/2/hi/health/3355751.stm

Held, D. and McGrew, A. (2007). *Globalization Theory.* Cambridge: Polity Press.

Hessler, K. (2008). 'Exploring the Philosophical Foundations of the Human Rights Approach to International Public Health Ethics'. In M. Boylan (ed.), *International Public Health Policy and Ethics* (pp. 31–43). New York: Springer.

Hogan, M. C., Foreman, K. J., Naghavi, M., Ahn, S. Y., Wang, M., Makela, S. M. and Murray, C. J. (2010). 'Maternal Mortality for 181 Countries, 1980–2008: A Systematic Analysis of Progress towards Millennium Development Goal 5'. *Lancet*, 375(9726), 1609–23.

Hogg, R. S., O'Shaughnessy, M. V., Gataric, N., Yip, B., Craib, K., Schechter, M. T., and Montaner, J. S. (1997). 'Decline in Deaths from AIDS due to New Antiretrovirals'. *Lancet*, 349(9061), 1294.

Hogg, R. S., Heath, K. V., Yip, B., Craib, K. J., O'Shaughnessy, M. V., Schechter, M. T. and Montaner, J. S. (1998). 'Improved Survival among HIV-infected Individuals following Initiation of Antiretroviral Therapy'. *Journal of the American Medical Association*, 279(6), 450–4.

Hogg, R. S., Yip, B., Chan, K. J., Wood, E., Craib, K. J. P., O'Shaughnessy, M. V.

and Montaner, J. S. (2001). 'Rates of Disease Progression by Baseline CD4 Cell Count and Viral Load after Initiating Triple-drug therapy'. *Journal of the American Medical Association*, 286(20), 2568–77.

Hollis, A. and Pogge, T. (2008). *The Health Impact Fund, Making New Medicines Accessible for All: A Report of Incentives for Global Health*. Incentives for Global Health.

Horsman, J., Furlong, W., Feeny, D. and Torrance, G. (2003). 'The Health Utilities Index (HUI): Concepts, Measurement Properties and Applications'. *Health and Quality of Life Outcomes*, 1(54), 1–13.

Horton, R. (2010). 'The Continuing Invisibility of Women and Children'. *Lancet*, 375(9730), 1941–3.

House of Commons Select Committee on Health (2005). *Third Report*. London: House of Commons.

Hurst, S. (2008). 'Vulnerability in Research and Health Care; Describing the Elephant in the Room? *Bioethics*, 22(4), 191–202.

Hyder, A. H. and Morrow, R. H. (1999). 'Steady State Assumptions in DALYs: Effect on Estimates of HIV Impact'. *Journal of Epidemiology and Community Health*, 53(1), 43–5.

IASC (2006). 'Women, Girls, Boys and Men. Different Needs – Equal Opportunities. Gender Handbook'. *Humanitarian Action*.

International Federation of Red Cross and Red Crescent Societies (1965). *Proclamation of the Fundamental Principles of the Red Cross*. Vienna: IFRC.

International Conference of the Red Cross and Red Crescent Societies (1994). *Code of Conduct for The International Red Cross and Red Crescent Movement and NGOs in Disaster Relief*. Geneva: IFRC.

International Monetary Fund (2011). List of countries by GDP (PPP) per capita, from http://en.wikipedia.org/wiki/List_of_countries_by_GDP_%28PPP%29_per_capita#cite_note-0

International Organization for Migration (2005). *World Migration 2005: Costs and Benefits of International Migration* (Vol. 3).

Jacobs, L. (1996). 'Can an Egalitarian Justify Universal Access to Health Care?' *Social Theory and Practice* 22, 315–48.

Jaggar, A. M. (2002). 'A Feminist Critique of the Alleged Southern Debt'. *Hypatia*, 17(4), 119–42.

James, P. D., Wilkins, R., Detsky, A. S., Tugwell, P. and Manual, D. G. (2007). 'Avoidable Mortality by Neighbourhood Income in Canada: 25 Years after the Establishment of Universal Health Insurance'. *Journal of Epidemiology and Community Health*, 61, 287–96.

Jamison, D., Breman, J., Measham, A., Alleyne, G., Claeson, M., Evans, D., Jha, P., Mills, A. and Musgrove, P. (2006). *Disease Control Priorities in Developing Countries*. Washington, DC: The World Bank and Oxford University Press.

Jenkins, S. P. (1999). POVDECO: Stata module to calculate poverty indices

with decompositon by subgroup, from http://ideas.repec.org/c/boc/bocode/
s366004.html

Johnston, K. M., Levy, A. R., Lima, V. D., Hogg, R. S., Tyndall, M. W.,
Gustafson, P. and Montaner, J. S. (2010). 'Expanding Access to HAART:
A Cost-effective Approach for Treating and Preventing HIV'. *Aids*, 24(12),
1929–35.

Johri, M. and Ako-Arrey, D. (2011). 'The Cost-effectiveness of Preventing
Mother-to-child Transmission of HIV in Low- and Middle-income
Countries: Systematic Review'. *Cost Effectiveness and Resource Allocation*,
9(3).

Joint Canada/United States Survey of Health (2004). *Findings and Public Use
Microdata File*.

Jones, P. (1994). *Rights*. Oxford: MacMillan.

Jonsen, A. R. (1986). 'Bentham in a Box: Technology Assessment and Health
Care Allocation'. *Law, Medicine and Health Care*, 14(3–4), 172–4.

Justman, J., Koblavi-Deme, S., Tanuri, A., Goldberg, A., Gonzalez, L. F. and
Gwynn, C. R. (2009). 'Developing Laboratory Systems and Infrastructure
for HIV Scale-up: A Tool for Health Systems Strengthening in Resource-
limited Settings'. *Journal of Acquired Immune Deficiency Syndromes*, 52
Supplement 1, S30–33.

Kane, J. (1996a). 'Basal Inequalities – Reply'. *Political Theory*, 24, 401–6.

Kane, J. (1996b). 'Justice, Impartiality, and Equality: Why the Concept of
Justice Does Not Presume Equality'. *Political Theory*, 24, 375–93.

Kant, I. (1981). *Grounding for the Metaphysics of Morals* (J. Ellington, trans.).
Cambridge, MA: Hackett Publishing Co.

Kawachi, I., Subramanian, S. V. and Almeida-Filho, N. (2002). 'A Glossary
for Health Inequalities'. *Journal of Epidemiology and Community Health*, 56,
647–52.

Keith, R. (2007). 'Nurses on the Move – Review Essay'. *International Journal of
Health Planning and Management*, 22, 353–9.

Kind, P., Brooks, R. and Rabin, R. (2005). *EQ-5D Concepts and Methods: A
Developmental History*. Dordrecht: Springer.

King, C. H. and Bertino, A.-M. (2008). 'Asymmetries of Poverty: Why Global
Burden of Disease Valuations Underestimate the Burden of Neglected
Tropical Diseases'. *PLoS Neglected Tropical Disease*, 2(3), 209.

Kingma, M. (2006). *Nurses on the Move: Migration and the Global Health Care
Economy*. Ithaca, NY: Cornell University Press.

Kirigia, J. M., Gbary, A. R., Muthuri, L. K., Nyoni, J. and Seddoh, A. (2006).
'The Cost of Health Professionals' Brain Drain in Kenya'. *Biomed Central
Health Services Research*, 6(89).

Kittay, E. F. (1997). 'Human Dependency and Rawlsian Equality'. In D. T.
Meyers (ed.), *Feminists rethink the self*. Boulder, CO: Westview Press.

Kittay, E. F. (2002). 'Can Contractualism Justify State-supported Long-term Care Policies? Or, I'd Rather be Some Mother's Child. A reply to Nussbaum and Daniels'. *Ethical Choices in Long-term Care: What Does Justice Require?* Geneva: WHO.

Koivusalo, M. (2011). 'Trade and Health: The Ethics of Global Rights, Regulation and Redistribution'. In S. Benatar and G. Brock (eds), *Global Health and Global Health Ethics* (pp. 143–54). Cambridge: Cambridge University Press.

Krieger, N. and Birn, A. E. (1998). 'A vision of Social Justice as the Foundation of Public Health: Commemorating 150 Years of the Spirit of 1848'. *American Journal of Public Health*, 88, 1603–6.

Kymlicka, W. (2011). 'Citizenship in and Era of Globalization'. In G. W. Brown and D. Held (ed.), *The Cosmopolitanism Reader* (Vol. 435–441). Cambridge: Cambridge University Press.

Labonte, R., Schrecker, T., Packer, C. and Runnels, V. (2009). *Globalization and Health: Pathways, Evidence and Policy*. New York: Routledge.

Labonte, R. and Schrecker, T. (2011). 'The State of Global Health in a Radically Unequal World: Patterns and Prospects'. In S. Benatar and G. Brock (eds), *Global Health and Global Health Ethics* (pp. 24–36). Cambridge: Cambridge University Press.

Laher, F., Todd, C. S., Stibich, M. A., Phofa, R., Behane, X., Mohapi, L. and Gray, G. (2009). 'A Qualitative Assessment of Decisions Affecting Contraceptive Utilization and Fertility Intentions among HIV-positive Women in Soweto, South Africa'. *AIDS and Behavior*. (June; 13, Supplement 1), 47–54.

Lalonde, M. (1974). 'A New Perspective on the Health of Canadians'. *National Health and Welfare*. Government of Canada.

Laveist, T., Gaskin, D. and Trujillo, A. J. (2011). *Segregated Spaces, Risky Places: The Effects of Racial Segregation on Health Inequalities*. Washington, DC: Joint Center for Political and Economic Studies.

Laxminarayan, R., Chow, J. and Shahid-Salles, S. (2006). 'Intervention Cost-effectiveness: Overview of Main Messages'. In D. Jamison, J. Breman, A. Measham, G. Alleyne, M. Claeson, D. Evans, P. Jha, A. Mills and P. Musgrove (ed.), *Disease Control Priorities in Developing Countries* (pp. 35–86). Washington, DC: The World Bank and Oxford University Press.

Le Grand, J. (1991). *Equity and Choice: An Essay in Economics and Applied Philosophy*. London: HarperCollins Academic.

Lichtenberg, F. R. (2005). 'Pharmaceutical Innovation and the Burden of Disease in Developing and Developed Countries'. *Journal of Medicine and Philosophy* 30(6), 663–90.

Lopez, A., Ezzati, M., Jamison, D. and Murray, C. (2006). 'Measuring the Global Burden of Disease and Risk Factors, 1990–2001'. *Global Burden of Disease and Risk Factors* (pp. 1–13). Oxford: Oxford University Press.

Lopez, A., Mathers, C., Ezzati, M., Jamison, D. and Murray, C. (2006). 'Sensitivity and Uncertainty Analyses for Burden of Disease and Risk Factor Estimates'. In A. Lopez, M. Ezzati, D. Jamison and C. Murray (ed.), *Global Burden of Disease and Risk Factors*. Washington, DC: World Bank.

Lorenzo, F. M., Galvez-Tan, J., Icamina, K. et al. (2007). 'Nurse Migration from a Source Country Perspective: Philippine Country Case Study'. *Health Services Research*, 42(3, Part 2), 1406–18.

MacIntyre, S. (1997). 'The Black Report and Beyond: What are the Issues?' *Social Science and Medicine*, 44, 723–45.

Mahmudi-Azer, S. (2011). 'The International Arms Trade and Global Health'. In S. Benatar and G. Brock (eds), *Global Health and Global Health Ethics* (pp. 166–72). Cambridge: Cambridge University Press.

Malik, A. M. (2011). 'Denial of Flood Aid to the Ahmadiyya Muslim Community in Pakistan'. *Health and Human Rights*, 13(1), 1–8.

Mangham, L. J. and Hanson, K. (2008). 'Employment Preferences of Public Sector Nurses in Malawi: Results from a Discrete Choice Experiment'. *Tropical Medicine and International Health*, 13(12), 1433–41.

Mann, J. M. (1996). 'Health and Human Rights'. *British Medical Journal*, 312(7036), 924–5.

Mann, J. M. (1997). 'Medicine and Public Health, Ethics and Human Rights'. *The Hastings Center Report*, 27(3), 6–13.

Marchand, S., Wikler, D. and Landesman, B. (1998). 'Class, Health, and Justice. *The Milbank Quarterly*, 76(3), 449–67.

Marmot, M., Ryff, C. D., Bumpass, L. L., Shipley, M. and Marks, N. F. (1997). 'Social Inequalities in Health: Next Questions and Converging Evidence. *Social Science and Medicine*, 44, 901–10.

Marmot, M. and Wilkinson, R. G. (1999). *Social Determinants of Health*. Oxford: Oxford University Press.

Marmot, M. (2006). 'Health in an Unequal World: Social Circumstances, Biology and Disease'. *Clinical Medicine*, 6, 559–72.

Marmot, M. (2007). 'Achieving Health Equity: From Root Causes to Fair Outcomes'. *Lancet*, 370, 1153–63.

Marmot, M. (2008). 'Closing the Gap in a Generation: Health Equity through Action on the Social Determinants of Health'. *Lancet*, 372, 1661–9.

Marshall, T. H. (1952). *Citizenship and Social Class*. Cambridge: Cambridge University Press.

Massey, D. (2004). 'Geographies of Responsibility'. *Geografiska Annnaler*, 86, 5–18.

Massey, D. (2006). 'Space, Time, and Political Responsibility in the Midst of Global Inequality'. *Erdkunde*, 60(2), 89–95.

Mathers, C., Boerma, T. and Fat, D. M. (2008). *The Global Burden of Disease: 2004 Update*. Geneva: WHO.

McCoy, D., Bennett, S., Witter, S., Pond, B., Baker, B., Gow, J., Chand, S., Ensor, T. and McPake, B. (2008). 'Salaries and Incomes of Health Workers in sub-Saharan Africa'. *Lancet*, 371, 675–81.

McInnes, C. and Lee, K. (2006). 'Health, Security and Foreign Policy'. *Review of International Studies*, 32(1), 5–23.

McKie, J. and Richardson, J. (1982). 'The Rule of Rescue'. *Social Science and Medicine*, 56(12), 2407–19.

Michaud, C., Murray, C. and Bloom, B. (2001). 'Burden of Disease – Implications for Future Research'. *Journal of the American Medical Association*, 285(5), 535–9.

Miller, D. (1999). *Principles of Social Justice*. Cambridge, MA: Harvard University Press.

Miller, D. (2005). 'Against Global Egalitarianism'. *The Journal of Ethics*, 9(1–2), 55–79.

Miller, D. (2007). *National Responsibility and Global Justice*. Oxford: Oxford University Press.

Miller, D. (2008). 'Immigrants, Nations, and Citizenship'. *The Journal of Political Philosophy*, 16(4), 371–90.

Miller, S. C. (2009). 'Moral Injury and Relational Harm: Analyzing Rape in Darfur'. *Journal of Social Philosophy*, 40(4), 504–23.

Montaner, J., Hogg, R. S., Wood, E., Kerr, T., Tyndall, M., Levy, A. and Harrigan, P. R. (2006). 'The Case for Expanding Access to Highly Active Antiretroviral Therapy to Curb the Growth of the HIV Epidemic'. *Lancet*, 368(9534), 531–6.

Murray, C. (1994). 'Quantifying the Burden of Disease: The Technical Basis for Disability-adjusted Life Years'. *Bulletin of the World Health Organization*, 72(3), 429–45.

Murray, C. (1996). Rethinking DALYs. In C. Murray and A. Lopez (eds), *The Global Burden of Disease: A Comprehensive Assessment of Mortality and Disability from Diseases, Injuries and Risk Factors in 1990 and Projected to 2020* (pp. 1–98). Cambridge, MA: Harvard School of Public Health.

Murray, C., Salomon, J. and Mathers, C. (2000). 'A Critical Examination of Summary Measures of Population Health'. *Bulletin of the World Health Organization*, 78(8), 981–94.

Murray, C. and Lopez, A. (2000). 'Progress and Directions in Refining the Global Burden of Disease Approach: A Response to Williams'. *Health Economics*, 9, 68–89.

Murray, C. and Evans, D. (2003). 'Health Systems Performance Assessment: Goals, Framework and Overview'. In C. Murray and D. Evans (eds), *Health Systems Performance Assessment: Debates, Methods and Empiricism* (pp. 3–18). Geneva: WHO.

Murray, C. J. L. and Acharya, A. K. (1997). 'Understanding DALYs'. *Journal of Health Economics*, 16(6), 703–30.

Murray, C. J. L., Gakidou, E. E. and Frenk, J. (1999). 'Health Inequalities and Social Group Differences: What Should we Measure?' *Bulletin of the World Health Organization*, 77(7), 537–43.

Nagel, T. (2005). 'The Problem of Global Justice'. *Philosophy & Public Affairs*, 33(2), 113–47.

National Committee on Confidential Enquiries into Maternal Deaths (2003). *Saving Mothers 1999–2001*. Pretoria: Department of Health, South Africa.

Nickels, J. (2007). *Making Sense of Human Rights*. Oxford: Blackwell Publishing.

Nord, E., Pinto, J., Richardson, J., Menzel, P. and Ubel, P. A. (1999). 'Incorporating Societal Concerns for Fairness in Numerical Valuations of Health Programmes'. *Health Economics*, 8(1), 25–39.

Nord, E. (2002). 'My Goodness – And Yours: A History, and Some Possible Futures, of DALY Meanings and Valuation Procedures'. In C. Murray, J. Salomon, C. Mathers and A. Lopez (eds), *Summary Measures of Population Health: Concepts, Ethics, Measurement and Applications* (pp. 139–46). Geneva: WHO.

Nordenfelt, L. (2012). 'Standard Circumstances and Vital Goals: Comments on Venkatapurum's Critique'. *Bioethics*, available online early.

Nordenfelt, L., Khushf, G. and Fulford, K. W. M. (2001). *Health, Science, and Ordinary Language*. Amsterdam: Rodopi.

Norheim, O. F. and Asada, Y. (2009). 'The Ideal of Equal Health Revisited: Definitions and Measures of Inequity in Health Should be Better Integrated with Theories of Distributive Justice'. *International Journal for Equity in Health*, 8(1), 40.

Nunn, A. J., Mulder, D. W., Kamali, A., Ruberantwari, A., Kengeya-Kayondo, J.-F. and Whitworth, J. (1997). 'Mortality Associated with HIV-1 Infection over Five Years in a Rural Ugandan Population: Cohort Study'. *British Medical Journal*, 315, 767–71.

Nussbaum, M. (2000). *Women and Human Development: The Capabilities Approach*. Cambridge: Cambridge University Press.

Nussbaum, M. (2005). 'Beyond the Social Contract: Capabilities and Global Justice'. In G. Brook and H. Brighouse (eds), *The Political Philosophy of Cosmopolitanism* (Vol. 196–218). Cambridge: Cambridge University Press.

Nussbaum, M. (2005). 'Women's Bodies: Violence, Security, Capabilities'. *Journal of Human Development*, 6(2), 167–83.

Nussbaum, M. (2006). *Frontiers of Justice: Disability, Nationality, Species Membership*. Cambridge, MA: Belknap Press of Harvard University Press.

Nussbaum, M. (2011). *Creating Capabilities: The Human Development Approach*. Cambridge, MA and London: The Belknap Press of Harvard University Press.

OECD (2010). *International Migration of Health Workers: Improving International Cooperation to Address the Global Health Workforce Crisis.* Vienna: Organization for Economic Cooperation and Development.

O'Keefe, P., Westgate, K. and Wisner, B. (1976). 'Taking the Naturalness out of Natural Disasters'. *Nature*, 260(5552), 566–7.

Omran, A. R. (1971). 'The Epidemiologic Transition. A Theory of The Epidemiology of Population Change'. *The Milbank Quarterly*, 49, 509–38.

O'Neill, M. (2008). 'What Should Egalitarians Believe?' *Philosophy and Public Affairs*, 36, 119–56.

O'Neill, O. (1989). *Constructions of Reason: Explorations of Kant's Practical Philosophy.* Cambridge: Cambridge University Press.

O'Neill, O. (1996). *Towards Justice and Virtue.* Cambridge: Cambridge University Press.

O'Neill, O. (1998). 'Vulnerability and Finitude'. In E. Craig (ed.), *Routledge Encyclopedia of Philosophy.* London: Routledge.

O'Neill, O. (2005). 'The Dark Side of Human Rights'. *International Affairs*, 81(2), 427–39.

Orbinski, J. (2007). 'Global Health, Social Movements, and Governance'. In A. Cooper, F. Andrew, J. Kirton and T. Schrecker (eds), *Governing Global Health: Challenge, Response, Innovation* (pp. 29–40). Aldershot: Ashgate.

Ostlin, P. and Diderichsen, F. (2001). *Equity-oriented National Strategy for Public Health in Sweden.* Geneva: WHO.

Ottonelli, V. and Torresi, T. (2010). 'Inclusivist Egalitarian Liberalism and Temporary Migration: A Dilemma'. *Journal of Political Philosophy.*

Palella Jr, F. J., Delaney, K. M., Moorman, A. C., Loveless, M. O., Fuhrer, J., Satten, G. A. and Holmberg, S. D. (1998). 'Declining Morbidity and Mortality among Patients with Advanced Human Immunodeficiency Virus Infection. HIV Outpatient Study Investigators'. *New England Journal of Medicine*, 338(13), 853–60.

Palmer, D. (2006). 'Tackling Malawi's Human Resources Crisis'. *Reproductive Health Matters*, 14(27), 27–39.

Parekh, S. (2008). 'Care and Human Rights in a Globalized World'. *Southern Journal of Philosophy*, 46, 104–10.

Parfit, D. (1997). 'Equality and Priority'. *Ratio-New Series*, 10, 202–21.

Payne, S. (2006). *The Health of Men and Women.* Cambridge: Polity Press.

Penchansky, R. and Thomas, J. (1981). PThe Concept of Access: Definition and Relationship to Consumer SatisfactionP. *Medical Care*, 19(2), 127–40.

Perrin, M. E., Hagopian, A., Sales, A. and Huang, B. (2007). Nurse migration and its implications for Philippine Hospitals'. *International Nursing Review*, 54, 219–26.

Peter, F. and Evans, T. (2001). Ethical Dimensions of Health Equity. In T. Evans, M. Whitehead, F. Diderichsen, A. Bhuiya and M. Wirth (eds),

Challenging Inequities in Health: From Ethics to action. Oxford and New York: Oxford University Press.

Peterson, S. (2006). 'Epidemic Diseases and National Security'. *Security Studies*, 12(2), 43–81.

Pevnick, R. (2009). 'Social Trust and the Ethics of Immigration Policy'. *The Journal of Political Philosophy*, 17(2), 146–67.

Pinto, A. (2010). 'Denaturalizing "natural" Disasters: Haiti's Earthquake and the Humanitarian Impulse'. *Open Medicine*, 4(4).

Platform for International Cooperation on Undocumented Migrants (2007a). *Access to Health Care for Undocumented Migrants in Europe*. PICUM.

Platform for International Cooperation on Undocumented Migrants (2007b). *Undocumented Migrants – Symptom, Not the Problem*. PICUM.

Pogge, T. (2002a). *World Poverty and Human Rights*. Cambridge: Cambridge University Press.

Pogge, T. (2002b). *World Poverty and Human Rights: Cosmopolitan Responsibilities and Reforms*. Cambridge, MA: Polity Press.

Pogge, T. (2004). 'Relational Conceptions of Justice: Responsibilities for Health Outcomes'. In S. Anand, F. Peter and A. Sen (eds), *Public Health, Ethics, and Equity* (Vol. 135–161). Oxford: Oxford University Press.

Pogge, T. (2005a). 'Real World Justice'. *The Journal of Ethics*, 9, 29–53.

Pogge, T. (2005b). 'Severe Poverty as a Violation of Negative Duties'. *Ethics and International Affairs*, 19, 55–84.

Pogge, T. (2005c). 'Human Rights and Global Health: A Research Paradigm'. *Metaphilosophy*, 36(1–2), 182–209.

Pogge, T. (2007). 'Severe Poverty as a Human Rights Violation'. In T. Pogge (ed.), *Freedom from Poverty as a Human Right: Who Owes What to the Very Poor?* (pp. 16–18). Oxford: Oxford University Press.

Pogge, T. (2008a). 'Access to Medicines'. *Public Health Ethics*, 1(2), 73–82.

Pogge, T. (2008b). 'Healthcare Reform that Works for the US and the World's Poor'. *Global Health Governance*, 2.

Pogge, T. (2008c). *World Poverty and Human Rights*. Cambridge: Polity Press.

Pogge, T. (2010). 'Response to the Critics'. In A. Jaggar (ed.), *Thomas Pogge and his Critics* (pp. 175–243). Cambridge: Polity Press.

Pogge, T. (2011). 'The Health Impact Fund: How to Make New Medicines Accessible to All'. In S. Benatar and G. Brock (eds), *Global Health and Global Health Ethics* (pp. 241–50). Cambridge: Cambridge University Press.

Powers, M. and Faden, R. R. (2006). *Social Justice: The Moral Foundations of Public Health and Health Policy*. New York: Oxford University Press.

Preston, S. H. (2007). 'The Changing Relation between Mortality and Level of Economic Development' (reprinted from *Population Studies*, Vol. 29, July 1975). *International Journal of Epidemiology*, 36, 484–90.

Price-Smith, A. (2009). *Contagion and Chaos: Disease, Ecology, and National Security in the Era of Globalization*. Cambridge, MA: MIT Press.

Quinn, T. C. and Overbaugh, J. (2005). 'HIV/AIDS in Women: An Expanding Epidemic'. [Review]. *Science*, 308(5728), 1582–3.

Raghuram, P., Madge, C. and Noxolo. P. (2009). 'Rethinking Responsibility and Care for a Postcolonial World'. *Geoforum*, 40, 5–13.

Ramesh, R. (2008). 'India: Untouchables Suffer "Relief Discrimination" after Flood'. *The Guardian*, 3 September.

Rawls, J. (1971). *A Theory of Justice*. Cambridge, MA: The Belknap Press of Harvard University Press.

Rawls, J. (1993). *Political Liberalism*. New York: Columbia University Press.

Rawls, J. (1999). *The Law of Peoples; with, The Idea of Public Reason Revisited*. Cambridge, MA: Harvard University Press.

Raz, J. (1984). *The Morality of Freedom*. Oxford: Oxford University Press.

Raz, J. (2006). 'Human Rights in the New World Order'. *Columbia Public Law & Legal Theory Working Papers*, Paper 9175.

Raz, J. (2007). 'Human Rights Without Foundation'. *Oxford Legal Studies Research Paper* (No. 14).

Record, R. and Mohidin, A. (2006). 'An Economic Perspective on Malawi's Medical "Brain Drain"'. *Globalization and Health*, 2(12).

Redfield, P. (2005). 'Doctors, Borders and Life in Crisis'. *Cultural Anthropology*, 20(3), 328–91.

Refugee Council (2010). *Draft Response to Department of Health Consultation: Review of Access to NHS by Foreign Nationals*.

Reidpath, D. D., Allotey, P. A., Kouame, A. and Cummins, R. A. (2003). 'Measuring Health in a Vacuum: Examining the Disability Weight of the DALY'. *Health, Policy and Planning*, 18(4), 351–6.

Reynolds, L. (2002). *Poverty Alleviation through Participation in Fair Trade Coffee Networks: Existing Research and Critical Issues*.

Robinson, F. (2006). 'Ethical Globalization? States, Corporations, and the Ethics of Care'. In M. E. Hammington and Miller, D. C. (ed.), *Socializing Care*. Lanham, MD: Rowman and Littlefield.

Rochat, T., Richter, L., Doll, H., Buthelezi, N., Tomkins, A. and Stein, A. (2006). 'Depression among Pregnant Rural South African Women undergoing HIV Testing'. *Journal of the American Medical Association*, 295(12), 1376–8.

Rodriguez, R. M. (2008). 'The Labor Brokerage State and the Globalization of Filipina Care Workers'. *Signs*, 33, 794–9.

Rosa Dias, O. (2009). 'Inequality of Opportunity in Health: Evidence from a UK Cohort Study'. *Health Econ*, 18(9), 1057–74.

Rousseau. C., Ouimet, M.-J., ter Kuile, S., Kirmayer, L., Muñoz, M., Crépeau, F. and Nadeau, L. (2008). 'Health Care Access for Refugees and Immigrants with Precarious Status'. *Canadian Journal of Public Health,* 99(4), July–August, 290–2.

Ruger, J. P. (2006). 'Ethics and Governance of Health Inequalities'. *Journal of Epidemiology and Community Health,* 60(998–1002).

Ruger, J. P. (2010). *Health and Social Justice.* New York: Oxford University Press.

Rushton, S. (2011). 'Global Health Security: Security for Whom? Security for What'. *Political Studies,* 59(4), 779–96.

Salomon, J., Mathers, C., Chatterji, S., Sadana, R., Üstün, B. and Murray, C. (2003). 'Quantifying Individual Levels of Health: Definitions, Concepts, and Measurement Issues'. In C. Murray and D. Evans (ed.), *Health Systems Performance Assessment: Debates, Methods and Empiricism* (pp. 301–18). Geneva: WHO.

Salomon, J. and Murray, C. (2004). 'A Multi-method Approach to Measuring Health-state Valuations'. *Health Economics,* 13(3), 281–90.

Salomon, J. (2010). 'New Disability Weights for the Global Burden of Disease'. *Bulletin of the World Health Organization,* 88(12), 879–80.

Saul, J. (2005). *The Collapse of Globalism.* New York: Atlantic Books.

Scheffler, S. (1982). 'Natural Rights, Equality, and the Minimal State'. In J. Paul (ed.), *Reading Nozick.* Oxford: Basil Blackwell.

Scheffler, S. (2003a). 'What is Egalitarianism?' *Philosophy and Public Affairs,* 31, 5–39.

Scheffler, S. (2003b). *Boundaries and Allegiances: Problems of Justice and Responsibility in Liberal Thought.* Oxford: Oxford University Press.

Scheffler, S. (2005). 'Choice, Circumstances, and the Value of Equality'. *Politics, Philosophy and Economics,* 4, 5–28.

Schild, V. (2007). 'Empowering "Consumer-citizens" or Governing Female Subjects? The Institutionalization of "Self-development" in the Chilean Social Policy Field'. *Journal of Consumer Culture,* 7(2), 179–203.

Schroeder, D. and Gefenas, E. (2009). 'Vulnerability: Too Vague and Too Broad?' *Cambridge Quarterly of Healthcare Ethics,* 18, 113–21.

Schroeder, D. (2011). *Prevalence, Incidence, and Hybrid Approaches to Calculating DALYs.* Paper presented at the Critical Ethical Choices for DALYs meeting, The Institute for Health Metrics Evaluation.

Schwartz, L., Sinding, C., Hunt, M., Elie, L. Redwood-Campbell, L., Adelson, N., Luther, L., Ranford, J. and DeLaat, S. (2010). 'Ethics in Humanitarian Aid Work: Learning From the Narratives of Humanitarian Health Workers'. *American Journal of Bioethics Primary Research,* 1(3), 45–54.

Segall, S. (2009). *Health, Luck and Justice.* Princeton, NJ: Princeton University Press.

Selgelid, M. (2005). 'Ethics and Infectious Disease'. *Bioethics,* 19, 272–89.

Selgelid, M. (2008). 'A Full-pull Program for the Provision of Pharmaceuticals: Practical Issues'. *Public Health Ethics,* 1(2), 134–45.

Selgelid, M. (2011). 'Justice, Infectious Diseases and Globalization'. In S. Benatar and G. Brock (eds), *Global Health and Global Health Ethics* (pp. 89–96). Cambridge, MA: Cambridge University Press.

Sen, A. (1981). 'Rights and Agency'. *Philosophy and Public Affairs*, 2, 3–39.

Sen, A. (1982a). 'Equality of What?' In S. M. Press (ed.), *Choice, Welfare, and Measurement*. Cambridge: MIT Press.

Sen, A. (1982b). *Welfare and Measurement* (2nd edition). Cambridge, MA: Harvard University Press.

Sen, A. (1992). *Inequality Reexamined*. Cambridge, MA: Harvard University Press.

Sen, A. (1996). 'On the Status of Equality'. *Political Theory*, 24, 394–400.

Sen, A. (1997a). *On Economic Inequality* (expanded edition with a substantial annexe by J. E. Foster and A. Sen, eds). Oxford: Oxford University Press.

Sen, A. (1997b). *Resources, Values and Development*. Cambridge, MA: Harvard University Press.

Sen, A. (1998). 'Mortality as an Indicator of Economic Success and Failure'. *The Economic Journal*, 108, 1–25.

Sen, A. (2002). 'Why Health Equity'? *Health Economics*, 11, 659–66.

Sen, A. (2009). *The Idea of Justice*. London: Allen Lane.

Shue, H. (1996). *Basic Rights: Subsistence, Affluence and US Foreign Policy* (2nd edition). Princeton, NJ: Princeton University Press.

Singer, P. (2004). *One World: The Ethics of Globalization*. New Haven, CT and London: Yale University Press.

Smits, J. and Monden, C. (2009). 'Length of Life Inequality around the Globe'. *Social Science and Medicine*, 68(6), 1114–23.

Snyder, J. (2009). 'Is Health Worker Migration a Case of Poaching?' *The American Journal of Bioethics*, 9(3), 3–7.

Soja, E. (1989). *Postmodern Geographies: The Reassertion of Space in Critical Social Theory*. London: Verso.

South African Department of Health (2011). 'Database of Medicine Prices', from http://www.doh.gov.za/department/pee/03Aug2011.zip

Sreenivasan, G. (2007). 'Health Care and Equality of Opportunity'. *Hastings Center Report*, 37(2), 21–31.

StataCorp. (2009). 'Stata Statistical Software: Release 11.0'. College Station, TX.

Steinbrook, R. (2002). 'Nursing in the Crossfire'. *New England Journal of Medicine*, 346, 1757–66.

Stemplowska, Z. (2009). 'Making Justice Sensitive to Responsibility'. *Political Studies*, 57(2), 237–59.

Stilwell, B., Diallo, K., Zurn, P. et al. (2004). 'Migration of Health Care Workers from Developing Countries: Strategic Approaches to its Management'. *Bulletin of the World Health Organization*, 82, 595–600.

Stuckler, D., King, L., Robinson, H. and McKee, M. (2008). 'WHO's Budgetary Allocations and Burden of Disease: A Comparative Analysis'. *Lancet*, 372(9649), 1563–9.

Sudhir, A., Peter, F. and Sen, A. (2006). *Public Health, Ethics, and Equity*. Oxford: Oxford University Press.

Tan, K.-C. (2004). *Justice without Borders: Cosmopolitanism, Nationalism and Patriotism*. Cambridge: Cambridge University Press.

Tan, K.-C. (2008). A Defense of Luck Egalitarianism. *Journal of Philosophy*, 11, 665–90.

Temkin, L. (1993). *Inequality*. Oxford: Oxford University Press.

Temkin, L. (2003). 'Egalitarianism Defended'. *Ethics*, 113, 764–82.

Terry, F. (2002). *The Paradox of Humanitarian Action: Condemned to Repeat*. Ithaca, NY: Cornell University Press.

The Global Fund (2010). Regional Price Reference, from http://bi.theglobalfund. org/analytics/saw.dll?Dashboard&nqUser=PQRExternalUser&PQRLAN GUAGE=en&PortalPath=/shared/PQR%20External%20Users/_portal/ PQR%20Public&Page=Regional%20Price%20Reference

'The Humanitarian Charter and Minimum Standards in Disaster Response' (2000), from http://www.sphereproject.org

The Royal College of General Practitioners (2009). *Position Statement: Failed Asylum Seekers/ Vulnerable Migrants and Access to Primary Care*. London.

Thomson, R. G. (2010). *What can Disability Studies do for Bioethics?* Paper presented at the International Network for Feminist Approaches to Bioethics, Singapore.

Tolentino, R. B. (1996). 'Bodies, Letters, Catalogs: Filippinas in Transnational Space'. *Social Text*, 48 (Autumn), 49–76.

Tronto, J. (2003). *Moral Boundaries*. New York: Routledge.

Tronto, J. (2006). 'Vicious Circles of Privatized Caring'. In M. E. Hamington and D. C. Miller (eds), *Socializing Care*. Lanham, MD: Rowman and Littlefield.

Trouiller, P., Torreele, E., Olliaro, P., White, N., Foster, S., Wirth, D. and Pécoul, B. (2002). 'Drugs for Neglected Diseases: A Failure of the Market and a Public Health Failure?' *Tropical Medicine and International Health 2002*, 945–51.

UNICEF (2004) 'Children on the Brink 2004: A Joint Report of New Orphan Estimates and a Framework for Action'. At: www.unicef.org/publications/ cob_layout6-013.pdf

United Nations (1948). 'The Universal Declaration of Human Rights', from http://www.un.org/en/documents/udhr/index.shtml

United Nations (1966). *International Covenant on Economic, Social and Cultural Rights* (Vol. 993). New York: UN.

United Nations (1986). 'Age Structure of Mortality in Developing Countries', from http://www.un.org/esa/population/publications/Age_Structure_of_

Mortality/Age_Structure.htm UNAIDS (2010). *Global Report: UNAIDS Report on the Global AIDS Epidemic 2010*. Geneva: UNAIDS.

United Nations Development Programme (2010). *The Human Development Report 2010: Technical Notes*. New York: UN Development Programme.

UNICEF (2011). 'Levels & Trends in Child Mortality – Report 2011'.

United Nations Millennium Declaration (2000). New York: UN

United Nations (2001). 'Millennium Development Goals', from http://www.un.org/millenniumgoals/

United Nations (2009). *The Millennium Development Goals Report 2009*. New York: UN.

United Nations Millennium Development Goals (2010). *2010 Malawi Millennium Development Goals Report*. New York: UNDP.

Üstün, T., Rehm, J., Chatterji, S., Saxena, S., Trotter, R., Room, R. et al. (1999). 'Multiple-informant Ranking of the disabling effects of Different Health Conditions in 14 Countries'. *Lancet*, 354 (9173), 111–15.

Venkatapuram, S. (2009). 'Epidemiology and Social Justice in Light of Social Determinants of Health'. *Bioethics*, 23, 78–89.

Venkatapuram, S., Bell, R. and Marmot, M. (2010). 'The Right to Sutures: Social Epidemiology, Human Rights, and Social Justice'. *Health and Human Rights. An International Journal*, 12(2).

Venkatapuram, S. (2011a). *Health Justice. An Argument from the Capabilities Approach*. Cambridge: Polity Press.

Venkatapuram, S. (2011b). 'Nussbaum's Capabilities Theory and Health Policy'. In B. Hawa and N. Weidtmann (eds), *The Capability Approach On Social Order*. Munster: LIT Verlag.

Venkatapuram, S. (2012). 'Health, Vital Goals and Central Human Capabilities'. *Bioethics*, available online entry.

Vertovec, S. and Cohen, R. (2002). *Conceiving Cosmopolitanism: Theory, Context and Practice*. Oxford: Oxford University Press.

Voigt, K. (2007). 'The Harshness Objection: Is Luck Egalitarianism Too Harsh on the Victims of Option Luck?' *Ethical Theory and Moral Practice*, 10(3), 389–407.

Waage, J., Banerji, R. and Campbell, O. (2010). 'The Millennium Development Goals: A Cross-sectoral Analysis and Principles for Goal-setting after 2015'. *Lancet*, 376, 991–1023.

Walton, D. A., Farmer, P. E., Lambert, W., Léandre, F., Koenig, S. P. and Mukherjee, J. S. (2005). 'Integrated HIV Prevention and Care Strengthens Primary Health Care: Lessons from Rural Haiti'. *Journal of Public Health Policy*, 25(2), 137–58.

Wasserman, D. (2006). 'Disability, Capability, and Thresholds for Distributive Justice'. In A. Kaufman (ed.), *Capabilities Equality: Basic Issues and Problems*. New York and London: Routledge.

Weiss, T. G. (1999). 'Principles, Politics, and Humanitarian Action'. *Ethics and International Affairs*, 13(1), 1–22.

Wellman, C. H. and Cole, P. (2011). *Debating the Ethics of Immigration: Is There a Right to Exclude?* Oxford: Oxford University Press.

Wenar, L. (2005). 'The Nature of Human Rights'. In A. Follesdal and T. Pogge (eds), *Real World Justice: Grounds, Principles, Human Rights and Social Institutions* (pp. 285–94). Dordrecht: Springer.

Whitehead, M. (1990). *The Concepts and Principles of Equity in Health.* Copenhagen: WHO Regional Office for Europe.

Whitehead, M. (1992). 'The Concepts and Principles of Equity and Health'. *International Journal of Health Services*, 22(3), 429–45.

WHO Commission on Social Determinants of Health (2008). 'Closing the Gap in a Generation: Health Equity through Action on the Social Determinants of Health'. *Final Report of the Commission on Social Determinants of Health.* Geneva: WHO.

Wikipedia (2011). List of Countries by Life Expectancy, from http://en.wikipedia.org/wiki/List_of_countries_by_life_expectancy#List_by_the_United_Nations_.282005-2010.29

Wikler, D. and Brock, D. W. (2007). 'Population-level Bioethics: Mapping a New Agenda'. In A. Dawson and M. Verweij (eds), *Ethics, Prevention, and Public Health* (pp. 78–94). New York: Oxford University Press.

Wilkinson, R. G. and Pickett, K. (2009). *The Spirit Level: Why More Equal Societies Almost Always do Better.* London: Allen Lane.

Williams, A. (1997). 'Intergenerational Equity: An Exploration of the "Fair Innings" Argument'. *Health Economics*, 6(2), 117–32.

Williams, A. (1999). 'Calculating the Global Burden of Disease: Time for a Strategic Reappraisal?' *Health Economics*, 8(1), 1–9.

Williams, A. (2000). 'Comments on the Response by Murray and Lopez'. *Health Economics*, 9(1), 83–6.

Wimmer, A. and Glick-Schiller, N. (2002). 'Methodological Nationalism and Beyond: Nation Building, Migration, and the Social Sciences'. *Global Networks*, 2(4), 301–34.

Wolbring, G. (2011). 'Disability, Displacement and Public Health: A Vision for Haiti'. *Canadian Journal of Public Health*, 102(2), 157–9.

Woodward, D. (2005). 'The GATS and Trade in Health Services: Implications for Health Care in Developing Countries'. *Review of International Political Economy*, 12(3).

Woodward, J. (1992). 'Commentary: Liberalism and Migration'. In B. Barry and R. E. Goodin (eds), *Free Movement: Ethical Issues in the Transnational Migration of People and of Money.* London and New York: Harvester Wheatsheaf.

World Bank (2009). *Remittance Data.* Washington, DC: World Bank.

World Health Organization (1948). *Constitution of World Health Organization.* Geneva: WHO.

World Health Organization (2000). *World Health Report 2000. Health Systems: Improving Performance.* Geneva: WHO.

World Health Organization (2002a). *Gender and Health in Disasters.* Geneva: WHO Department of Gender and Women's Health.

World Health Organization (2002b). *World Health Report: Reducing Risks, Promoting Healthy Life.* Geneva: WHO.

World Health Organization (2004a). *Death and DALY Estimates for 2004 by Cause for WHO Member States.* Geneva: WHO.

World Health Organization (2004b). *World Health Report 2004.* Geneva: WHO.

World Health Organization (2006a). *Country Health System Fact Sheet 2006 Malawi.* Geneva: WHO.

World Health Organization (2006b). *World Health Report 2006: Working Together for Health.* Geneva: WHO.

World Health Organization (2007). *World Health Statistics.* Geneva: WHO.

World Health Organization (2009a). *The Nursing Community, Macroeconomic and Public Finance Policies: Towards a Better Understanding.* Geneva: WHO.

World Health Organization (2009b). *Towards Universal Access: Scaling up Priority HIV/AIDS Interventions in the Health Sector – Progress Report 2009.* Geneva: WHO.

World Health Organization (2010a). *Global Report on Antimalarial Drug Efficacy and Drug Resistance: 2000–2010.* Geneva: WHO.

World Health Organization (2010b). *Towards Universal Access: Scaling up Priority HIV/AIDS Interventions in the Health Sector – Progress Report 2010.* Geneva: WHO.

World Health Organization (2010c). *Trends in Maternal Mortality: 1990 to 2008.* Geneva: WHO.

World Health Organization (2011a). *Global Atlas of the Health Workforce.* Geneva: WHO.

World Health Organization (2011b). *Regional Burden of Disease Estimates for 2004.* Geneva: WHO.

Youde, J. (2005). 'Enter the Fourth Houseman: Health Security and International Relations Theory'. *Whitehead Journal of Diplomacy and International Relations,* 6(1), 193–208.

Young, I. M. (2000). *Inclusion and Democracy.* Oxford: Oxford University Press.

Young, I. M. (2004). 'Responsibility and Global Labor Justice'. *Journal of Political Philosophy,* 12(4), 365–88.

Young, I. M. (2006). 'Responsibility and Global Justice: A social connection model'. *Social Philosophy and Policy,* 23, 102–30.

Young, I. M. (2007). *Global Challenges: War, Self-Determination and Responsibility for Justice.* Cambridge: Polity Press.

INDEX

Note: page numbers in *italics* denote figures or tables